SO-DFH-706

Get Your Head Out of the Fridge!

HOW TO STOP BEING A FOODAHOLIC

Dr. JERRY L. WALKE
with Angela Y. Whitt, R.N.

originally titled *Confronting and Conquering Foodaholism*

A Perigee Book

Perigee Books
are published by
The Putnam Publishing Group
200 Madison Avenue
New York, NY 10016

Library of Congress Cataloging-in-Publication Data

Walke, Jerry L.
    Get your head out of the fridge.

    Reprint. Originally published: Confronting and
conquering foodaholism. Jackson, Ohio: Liberty
Press, c1985.
    1. Reducing—Psychological aspects.
2. Obesity—Psychological aspects.   3. Food habits.
I. Whitt, Angela Y.   II. Walke, Jerry L.
Confronting and conquering foodaholism.   III. Title.
RM222.2.W256   1987   613.2'5'019   86-30427
ISBN 0-399-51370-1

Previously published in a limited edition under the title
Confronting and Conquering Foodaholism

Printed in the United States of America

1 2 3 4 5 6 7 8 9 10

DEDICATION

This book is dedicated to two very special people. Katharine Walke Emery, my loyal daughter, is an aspiring novelist and poet whose articulateness and "word pictures" are already far beyond any abilities I've ever possessed. If she does not become a best-selling novelist, it will either be because she isn't writing it or the right people aren't reading it.

Angela Yvonne Whitt, registered nurse, who inspired both my writing of this book and many of the ideas in it—particularly in the areas of nutrition, grooming, and dress. Ms. Whitt, who is also a model, has been the major influence of my return to writing and publishing. I'm forever in her debt.

ACKNOWLEDGMENTS

I would like to pay tribute to my family members, both living and deceased, for their contributions to my life—and my knowledge of obsessive-compulsive eating (foodaholism). A large percentage of them, including my late father, were foodaholics. Therefore, unfortunately, much of my learning was both painful and negative. Yet, they are (and were) all very good, hardworking people who serve community, country, and humanity in general. I'm most proud of all of them.

A special thanks to my typist and word processor, Lisa Cawthorne. She has been invaluable and every writer needs a person of her special talents. Ms. Cawthorne is a beautiful and enterprising woman who aspires to business entrepreneurship—and she's already well on her way at a youthful age.

ARE YOU READY FOR THIS BOOK?

A few years ago, I noticed a long line of people in a large shopping mall. I walked ahead to see their destination and discovered they were waiting to step on some new-fangled, computerized scales that *announced* your weight over a small loudspeaker.

I was intrigued, also, and went back to stand in the relatively quick-moving line. As I neared the scales, I could hear the robot-ish voice saying, "102 lbs., thank you, little boy; 136 lbs., thank you, ma'am; 184 lbs., thank you sir." Soon it was my turn. I stepped on gingerly and the speaker blared defiantly, "ONE AT A TIME, PLEASE!"

I knew then that it was time to start my program and write this book. If you think you might receive equal wrath from those untactful scales, then you're ready to read this book.

(The above story is gratefully dedicated to the late and rotund Bill Hess, Head Football Coach at Ohio University. I so admired him and heard him tell this banquet joke many times).

FOREWORD

I have taken careful steps to make this book concise, easy to read, and as brief as possible. In addition, I attempt to write in a manner that makes you, the reader, feel as though I am actually talking with you personally. This, in my opinion, is the essence of both good teaching and good writing. I sincerely hope you will feel I have accomplished all this as you read on. Keep in mind that just because you don't like what I'm saying at given times does not mean it may not be true!

I have spent the past ten years in in-depth study of self-concept psychology and how it relates to obesity, obsessive-compulsive eating, and foodaholism. I've also conducted extensive obesity counseling for both adults and children. In addition, I've studied diligently how successful people think and live. This book is a culmination of all my work. It is my true desire that your life is enriched by reading it.

— TABLE OF CONTENTS —

PART I

LET'S
DISCUSS
OBESITY

CHAPTER ONE

Obesity In Contemporary Society

"Have You No Compassion, Dr. Walke?"

Recently, I asked a student to read the beginning portions of the manuscript of this book and invited her critique. The woman, Dorothy, is a conscientious and intelligent student in her 30's and I value her opinion. She is also a very over-weight woman and certainly a foodaholic. In addition, she is a very good woman; struggling and seeking identity; desiring to both give and receive compassion; and somewhat a "fan" of yours truly. Hence, my invitation of her criticism.

She read the first ten pages and then wrote me this strong note: "You must mix in some compassion before readers like me drown in pain!"

This brief critique was actually quite astute and observant, so I wrote her the following reply: "Dorothy, you will discover if you examine the remainder of my manuscript closely, that most of my book is highly compassionate. Indeed, I wrote this book in the first place because of compassion for the true "hooked" foodaholic. I have spent most of my life as one and the past ten years observing, studying, and working with them (and myself). I have witnessed first-hand their burden and tragic-ness within my own family. My closest cousin, Diane, a brilliant English teacher, died at 31 years old mainly due to food abuse. My father, my aunts and uncles, my grandparents—it was everywhere. Many times I cried (and still do) over their plight—and my own. This book IS compassion!

At the same time, compassion, especially in the beginning phase, will not help conquer foodaholic-ism. The obsessive-compulsive eater must first CONFRONT his problem and realize that it is a deep-seeded, imbedded/internalized, psychological and emotional problem. He/she must be "bopped on the head!" This usually requires getting tough with them and that's just what I intend to do—out of pure compassion!

This is a hard-hitting book. If the shoe fits, wear it, lest no article of clothing you have will ever fit!

OBESITY IN THE U.S.—AND WORLD!

Obviously, obesity is an awesome problem in this country today—and in many other countries throughout the world. Millions of people are literally "grossly overweight."—that is, weighing at least 30 pounds or more than they should. And even though psychologists largely understand the reasons, this widespread obesity is tragic—and inexcusable!

Gross obesity is by far the worst health problem in the world today. Nothing else touches it except, very ironically, gross starvation. Unfortunately, the two problems are inter-connected and "feed" off one another. I'll discuss this in greater detail soon.

Our society moralizes and frets about alcohol abuse, drug abuse, cancer, child abuse, etc. We are bombarded with statistics showing the destruction they wrought. All well and good, yet we are not informed properly that the abuse of food is by far the major crippler and killer of human beings on this earth today—probably even surpassing war. We unnecessarily eat ourselves into premature heart attacks, strokes, diabetes, high blood pressure, stress, anxiety attacks and poor mental health. Yes, obesity almost always causes some form of conscious or unconscious poor self-concept and reduced mental health through inadequate coping strategies.

We receive a fantastic variety of food advertising and commercials through our news media each minute, hour, and day. Though well-meaning—and part of our culture and economic system—they almost all have the same message of "Eat more food, eat more food, eat yourself to death."

I chuckle (or cry) when I hear moralistic preaching that "too much alcohol, or pot smoking, or some other drug will cause brain damage." Those people should be told that by far the major cause of "brain damage" to the human animal today is the abuse of food substances. Nothing else even comes near food as the eventual chief destructor of the human circulatory system, and therefore, the brain.

THE OBESITY-STARVATION IRONY

We, the U.S. of A., are one of the world's "fat-cat" nations. We are one of the few peoples who have to stand in line to get OUT of supermarkets and restaurants rather than to just get IN to find something (anything!) to eat. We are quite fortunate. Yet, like all good fortune, we pay a price. American diet habits are the classic example of "there is no such thing as a free lunch." We pay, sooner or later, health-wise and monetarily (drug and doctor bills).

In this country, most people eat twice as much daily as they need to live healthfully. At the same time, most also eat five times as much as they need to live healthfully. I'll solve this "double-talk" riddle for you in a few minutes.

The price we pay for our abundant food supply is twofold:

1) The almost endless number of both physical and mental health problems that "grow" out of obsessive-compulsive eating. (Has it occurred to you that we would not have a doctor shortage here; medical costs would not be out of control; and a high percentage of physicians would not be so highly wealthy were it not for our abundant food supply and our obsession with eating it all. "Clean your plate, child!")

Many of these resulting health problems are not evident unless you look closely. For example, that most people who suffer back ailments are overweight and the combination of big belly, gravity, and lack of exercise (muscle-tone) causes a disc to slip. This little scenario is one of the major reasons both your local orthopedic surgeon and your local chiropractor drive Mercedes. Furthermore, add the millions of people who suffer poor self-concept and all the emotional-social problems that accompany poor self-image—from shyness to stress, from depression to anxiety, from anti-social behavior to withdrawal, ad infinitum. And much research shows that over

90% of grossly over-weight people do suffer from very poor self-concept, whether or not they admit it to themselves or others. I'll discuss this in detail later.

2) The collective guilt that we Americans (especially knowledgable ones and/or humanistic and Christian ones) have to feel as we learn that our "fat-catness"—along with the other fat-cat nations—is a major cause of world starvation. IF we all ate only what it took to live very healthfully, there would be more than enough food supply for the world's human horde mass—at least at this time. But we truly do "want our cake and eat it too." That is, we want to have the freedom to eat any darn thing we please, have plenty more where that came from (in the pantry), and yet want to feel humane and help the starving.

So we ease our guilt by either a) "praying about it"; b) sending a few dollars to some helping organization; or c) going to our well-stocked pantry and getting a can of something we don't like anyway, (kale, spinach, etc.) and carrying it to the church basement for a Care package drive for Ethiopians. And then it's off to get our two Big Macs, milkshake and "keep our eyes on our fries." All the while feeling so smugly that "I've done my part!"

Allow me a quick social-moral message. I truly believe that if Jesus Christ were bodily walking this earth today, he would be spending almost fulltime crusading against world starvation and against our "fat-catness." I further believe that any "Christian" church worthy of its name must be doing the same. I believe this so strongly that it is the major reason I am writing this section of the book; that I do personal counseling in these areas; that I hold seminars; that I cured myself of foodaholic-ism; and that I, too, am quickly becoming a "crusader" against world starvation and for "eating only what you need to live healthfully, my fellow human."

A NOTE TO THE CLERGY

It is not the purpose of this book to repeatedly bring out obesity and obsessive-compulsive eating as a moral and ethical issue—though they obviously are. But to "harp" on it would not enhance the goals of this book and would probably even serve to weaken my efforts. So permit me to end this section with a rather strong note to ministers in the western world today. Nothing else touches the ravages over-eating produces—not cancer, not crime, not drugs, not alcohol, nothing!

Yet we listen every Sunday as thousands of ministers preach against all the "sin" in the world—including usually drugs, alcohol, crime, adultery, ad infinitum. Seldom do most of these ministers mention food abuse, and even when they do it is not done in a strong manner as are the other "sins" treated. Naturally, this is due to the fact that so many of their flock (who happen also to be donors to the donation plate) are grossly overweight and flat-out do not wish to be reminded. "Lay any guilt trip on me you want except that one, Reverend!"

But we must examine how man—and his church—has defined "sin" down through the ages. It's quite obvious that all "sin" has one common denominator: It consists of highly self-serving or self-satisfying (ego-centric) behavior and/or behavior that is destructive to others or self. Bingo! Obesity, overeating and obsessive-compulsive eating fit that self-indulgent bill as readily as ANY other "sin" you can come up with.

The nature of any religion is that each person must interpret his perception of its words, symbols, and leaders. In my mind, there is absolutely no doubt that if Jesus Christ were walking this earth to-day, one of the major thrusts of his ministry would be to crusade against world starvation and self-destruction through food. As already mentioned, the two are also closely related and Christ would recognize same.

C'mon ministers, rabbis, and priests, let's get serious about this whole thing!

Also, I have watched many members of my family, including my father, eat themselves into a premature grave—literally "gorge themselves to death"—and it was so painful to witness. I will discuss my loving and lovable father in detail to you later—for a specific reason.

But now quickly back to the double-talk riddle. Remember I said earlier that most Americans literally eat twice as much as they need to live healthfully. At the same time, most of them also eat five times as much as they need to live healthfully.

It's true. The answer lies in the fact that obese people often eat twice as many calories per day as they need to function very energetically. But, in addition, they eat much beef and pork. I wish to make no one angry, simply to state the truth when I say that the cow particularly is a highly wasteful meat machine. The various grains and legumes we use to force feed the cow in order to "build" your beef and steak for one meal would feed you five nutritious delicious meals, properly prepared. Ask any expert and he'll tell you I am correct—or darn close.

If I were king of the world—which I'm not and don't wish to be—only seldom would any human being be permitted to "pig out"—that is, eat far more than he needs to live quite healthfully. Though I wouldn't be too popular in my mother/home country, they'd love me in Ethiopia, Bangladesh, etc., wouldn't they?

One more point while I'm on my social soapbox, then we'll move on. Again let's take a look at our food advertising blitz in this country. Prime time TV; prime time for children (Saturday mornings); prime time for homemakers (daytime TV); in other words, almost continually, our food companies (rightfully so, in a free enterprise system) "condition" (advertise, propagandize) our people to the use of their products. They raise us from cradle to casket, from womb to tomb. The McDonald's "take-over" of Saturday morning cartoon time was legendary—and brilliant in Madison Avenue terms. It will go down in history as one of the great advertising campaigns in the history of mankind. They literally raised our children from pups and conditioned their tastebuds to McDonald's products. The manner is which they used the basic principles of behaviorism and behavioral engineering were nothing short of genius. Their influence of our youth (and soon to be adults) through positive reinforcement techniques like Ronald, Barry Manilow music; highly creative, catchy phrases; all-American imagery, etc. was behavioral modification at its best. To the point that now 19 million Americans enter McDonald's golden arches daily to eat a very average product. But in most of their customers' minds, mouths, stomachs, and tastebuds, their products are much more than my word "average."

But, back to the point, 90% of our food commercials, of which a great deal are beef-oriented, say these things (unwittingly) to our people:

A. Eat, eat, eat! Don't stop!

B. Eat more refined sugar!

C. Eat more grease and cholesterol! Hurry!

D. Clog up your arteries by the time you're 45 so we can do triple by-pass and make heart surgeons wealthy!

E. Have your only fun in life eating, bored person, so we can fit you for your casket as early as possible!

19

Make no mistake, the only reason for our longer life expectancy is advanced medicine through science. And, with that progress, add equal progress in dietary habits and we will find it commonplace for people to live to be 100 and be highly alert and active most of the way. We're heading to nursing homes much to early—thanks to abundant food supply and free enterprise promotion of same. Note here that I am not against free enterprise—in fact, love it. I'm only realistically describing the contemporary scene.

Now, simply to make a point, let's pretend that I had the financial resources to "take-over" prime time TV ad space for a while. I would create the following commercial (and ones similar) and bombard our people with it daily. The actors/actresses would be selected carefully, just as cunning Madison Avenue moguls presently "play the game":

The opening scene would show an American married couple. The man would be a very fat, obviously uncomfortable, unhappy, negative, almost despicable type character exiting a supermarket door. He would be pushing an over-loaded shopping cart brimming with every junk food item that could be placed in the cart. Various items such as cupcakes, cornchips, cheese dips, etc. would even be seen spilling over onto the pavement.

By his side would be an equally negative, equally despicable, highly obese "tub of grease" woman pushing another shopping cart loaded in the same manner—and spilling over the same way. (I am painting such an aggressively negative picture on purpose—not because of any PERSONAL axes to grind).

Trotting closely by their sides would be their young son and daughter—approximately eight years old and six years old. They, too, would be already very heavy, with obviously special-bought clothes draped over their sadly premature rolls of fat (why do so many mothers think that to fatten up their children proves "love" and good motherhood?) Every action of these two off-spring would also be carefully orchestrated to negatively reinforce the ad viewer. In short, they would exude pure disgustingness—whining, sniveling, over-indulged brats.

The children would be grabbing at the baskets and bleating such statements as "Mommy, I want some cupcakes now!"; "Daddy, open the cornchips now!" and "We want some candy!" The parents would be smacking their hands away and saying, "You kids can just wait until we get home" and "You can't be hungry, you just ate."

The children would be crying and screaming back at their parents that "No, we're hungry" and "We want to eat now" and grabbing items from the basket and ravenously tearing open wrappers. You may be thinking that this is exaggerated, but it will most certainly be repeated many times in America this very day.

Meanwhile, in the upper corner of the screen, I will create a different scenario:

Closely observing this entire "family food feud" will be a young Ethiopian mother and her son and daughter—same ages as the Americans. These people will also have been carefully chosen—all first being very skinny to the point of emaciation. However, they will be at the same time quite attractive, pleasant, appealing, and humble. (We love humility in America—especially when it consists of other people "giving in" to us).

The Ethiopian children will be holding their mother's hand, looking up at her in a pleading way, and saying in weakened voices, "Mother, we're so hungry, do we have anything to eat?" And "Why don't we have all we want to eat like those American children?"

The camera will pan close, show the mother's tears, anguish, and heartbreak as she says, "I know you're hungry, my children, but I have nothing. I don't really know why the Americans have so much—I guess it has a lot to do with technology, location geographically, and a little historical luck," and "Their parents have always taught them to share, but only in very small token ways. They mean well!"

Then the narrator will conclude the ad, "Many parents in this world tonight don't even know what they are going to feed their children tomorrow."

Remember, this commercial and others like it, will be repeated over and over on prime time, daytime, and Saturday mornings. If you don't think it will produce dramatic results, then you don't know human behavior very well. Oh sure, it won't affect Tessy Tubb maybe, or Oscar Obese, Freddy Fat, Max Macho, or Ralph Redneck. But, over a period of time, I'll get to the Jim Gentle's, the Chris Christian's, the Diane Do-Good's, the Reverend Right's, and hopefully even Billy Graham with all his clout. And surely all of the entertainers from the USA for Africa video will be affected. We will see very powerful movements against world starvation. We'll see it become very socially unpopular to be a "pigger-outer"—just as the past six years saw it become very un-chic to drive a "gas-hog car". Governmental reports will begin to show that we've reduced our food intake by 10%—then 20%, etc., just as we did with gasoline. Farmers will be reporting more surpluses for sale to under-nourished countries. Junk food companies will report lower earnings and start using their research and development expertise to create nourishing—yet tasty—snacks. The beef industry will stop mixing in so much fat and begin to prepare without grease (to their credit, many already are—just due to small pressures such as books like the one you are reading). Many churches, parental groups, and school "children" from kindergarten through college will lead the way. Other fat-cat nations will follow our lead (as usual). We'll find that we still have plenty to go around and most of us will be much healthier. The life expectancy will jump quickly and so will productivity—due to our increased vitality. Naturally, the Tessy Tubb's and the Oscar Obese's will still die quite early, going to their grave stating, "Well, everyone has to die some way" and "Eating is one of the few pleasures I get from life and if I can't pig-out, I might as well be dead." Pure, hybrid cop-out on life!

Special Note

No reader need take the above personally. It is a necessary scenario for you obsessive-compulsive eaters to understand. Let us continue. Hopefully, I'm getting your attention. There simply is no excuse for our present eating patterns in America. They are extremely over-indulgent and gravely destructive. We are too intelligent to embrace such culinary suicide.

LIVE TO BE 100 EASILY
AND HEALTHFULLY?

To emphasize the magnitude of the obesity problem in the "fat-cat" nations, I see no reason why most people should not be living to be a century old—and doing so quite alertly, given the vast knowledge of modern medicine. IF one reasonably monitors the substances which enter the body from the time of birth, such destructive maladies as heart attacks, strokes, high blood pressure, sugar diabetes, arteriosclerosis, gall bladder, etc. would become almost extinct. Sure, one still might get hit by a train, get maimed by a drunk or die of cancer, etc. However, I highly suspect that even many forms of cancer would decrease and can rationally philosophize that very possibly drunkeness and careless pulling out in front of trains would even decrease due to improved body chemistry.

CHAPTER TWO

Yes,
You Are A Foodaholic!

If you are grossly overweight, that is, if you weigh 30 pounds or more than you should reasonably weigh health-wise, then you are, in all probability, a foodaholic—an obsessive-compulsive eater. It would be rare that you weren't and, in that case, only a doctor could pinpoint your particular causal factor.

Psychologically, a foodaholic is exactly like an alcoholic in most every way (except, obviously, the degree of mind altering of alcohol). Actually, psychological profile wise, foodaholics are also similar to all other obsessive-compulsives (liars, gamblers, kleptomaniacs, etc.).

Many times in my classes a student will state emphatically, "Well, I just don't understand why anyone steals all the time and then says they can't help it." When I see that the person speaking is grossly overweight, I reply, "What do you mean you can't understand? Aren't you always saying that you're never going to overeat again? And aren't these statements most always made on a full stomach? And then when food is presented to you in the near future, don't you grab it up and stuff it down—and usually continue "ramrodding" it down even when your basic hunger pains are gone?"

After they admit this, I then say, "And then you have the nerve to chastise some person who truly doesn't want to steal (ring a bell?), and tells himself he won't this time (ring a bell?). But when something "tasty" is on the counter (ring a bell?) at K-Mart, he is driven to pick it up and put it in his mouth, (oops) pocket, (ring a bell?)." Beginning to see the profile?

The foodaholic is also like the alcoholic (and the other aforementioned), in that he can usually note the symptoms in others, but not himself (projection) and therefore cannot and/or will not admit to himself that he has a deep-seated problem (denial). And, also similarly, until he does so he is destined and doomed to wallow in his own problem (fat) until death do him part.

NOTE

Because I am male, I will write in the "he" gender rather than repeat he/she each time. Obesity is an equal problem in both men and women.

So, he travels through life, usually in "quiet desperation," believing that tomorrow he'll start a successful diet or that someday he'll be slender and trim like Frank Gifford, Robert Redford, Burt, Paul, etc. Tragically, he'll usually only ever become slender and REMAIN that way due to poor health caused by his gross overweightness. In other words, on his deathbed or in the nursing home, he probably will be just as trim as Tom Selleck is—but meanwhile, his prime years came, suffered, and went, and he has few good memories—except Thanksgiving and Christmas dinners, picnics, and special restaurants. And they were even accompanied by the stuffed, guilt "hangover" that followed. (Believe me, fellow foodaholics, writing this evokes 20 years of difficult, painful memories).

SO, HOW ABOUT DIETS?

Thousands of books, pamphlets, and magazine articles have been published over many years on every conceivable type of diet. Doctors, famous celebrities, military leaders, politicians, you name it, have created diets that "have worked for me and will work for you" or that "will make you beautiful just like Jane Fonda or Paul Newman." Millions of man hours have been spent and millions of dollars profitted. Ha, the National Enquirer alone has made a fortune on sales to foodaholics hoping for that final, ultimate diet that will restore their self-concept and lead them to earthly shangri-la.

What effect has all this had on the weight problem in this country? Almost none at all! What percentage of people have been helped, cured or changed? Almost nil! What "good" has been reaped? Minimal at most! Put quite simply, diets and diet programs in themselves are almost absolutely useless. It would be similar to putting an alcoholic accustomed to martinis on bloodymarys and beer. Of course, the foodaholic can't quit food all together but diet programs as such do little—usually nothing—to solve the true problem.

There have been various research projects conducted as to what percentage of people go on a concerted diet, lose a given amount of weight, and then have gained that weight back—plus more—one year later. Results vary some, but not too much. It is probably between 93%-97%, I'll settle for 95%. Think of it, 95 of every 100 persons simply cannot lose it and keep it off by dieting alone. The process of dieting in itself is a veritable waste of time. Why? The obsessive-compulsive need to eat has not been altered.

HOW ABOUT
CRASH AND "FAD" DIETS?

Most of you already know the answer. Useless and even dangerous. Dangerous for obvious health reasons (though I am a believer in periodic, organized fasting for different reasons than weight loss. I'll discuss later).

But there is a deeper reason that crash diets are useless—and it is related to why they are so popular. Obsessive-compulsive persons are marked by extreme, exaggerated, over-reactive, all-or-nothing behavior. So, when they eat, they "go all the way." And, you guessed it, when they diet they do the same. They "hit it hard" for a few days or few weeks, until they have lost a few pounds, sometimes many more. Little do they realize that their diet approach is nothing more than "practice" for their upcoming weight resurgence. Thus crash dieters literally lose thousands of pounds during their "elevator existence"—and gain thousands plus more. Their behavior is dismal to observe. I know because I watched them in my family all my life and spent many years "practicing" crash dieting as a way of life myself. It's just a long lonely road to nowhere. If you are a foodaholic reading this book earnestly and conscientiously, forget them.

HOW ABOUT PILLS?

I hope I'm insulting your intelligence to even have to cover this subject. NEVER, (and I seldom use that word) have I known a person who took "black beauties" or any other diet pill (speed) and lost weight effectively and then maintained same—except a few who then soon after had major health problems physically and/or emotionally. Though I cannot practice medicine, I find it difficult to believe that any physician who has even had a Psychology 101 course and understands anything at all about obsessive-compulsive eating would even prescribe them to a patient. I am both suspicious and leery of any doctor who does.

And though I know little about appetite supressants and how they work; and even though I could see they might have some merit as a "crutch" in the beginning steps of dietary habit change; I DO know that they could seldom serve any long-term purpose in effective weight loss.

HOW ABOUT
EXERCISE AND "WORKING OUT?"

Obviously, physical exercise is excellent, and as I'll discuss later, very beneficial and even essential. But there is a lot of misconception and misunderstanding about what exercise, as a means in itself, can do. It is vastly over-rated and many foodaholics spend much money in the belief that jazzercise, jogging, nautilus, health clubs, exercise apparatus, etc. will automatically make them slim and trim. This just does not happen—not until combined with learned dietary habit alteration. One might as well tell an alcoholic that he'll be "cured" if he exercises regularly, even if he heads for the bar or bottle after he sweats. However, as we'll see, exercise is necessary, and unfortunately, most foodaholics slowly but surely quit doing it.

HOW ABOUT WEIGHT WATCHERS
AND OTHER SIMILAR PROGRAMS?

I mentioned earlier that close to 95% of the people who go on a diet and lose a set number of pounds have gained it back plus more a year later. Therefore, only 5% are successful in maintaining their weight loss over a prolonged period. Actually, Weight Watchers, and other similar programs DO improve on this 5% figure—but not dramatically. The reason they do a little better is because they add, either knowingly or unknowingly, another dimension to weight loss and control, and it's admittedly a positive dimension. That is, they add the principles of a group therapy!

You see, the Weight Watchers program is mostly just another diet program. But their regular meetings, patterned strongly after Alcoholics Anonymous, serve to keep them watching out for and checking on each other. This camaraderie of fellow foodaholics is quite good and does eventually allow them to have a higher incidence of "successes" than most programs.

But, I repeat, not really a dramatically higher rate. As a trained counselor, I cannot and would not discount the great benefit of an ALLIED OTHER (friend, counselor, etc.) when one is attempting to alter behavior. However, Weight Watchers, in my opinion, falls short in two crucial areas:

1) Personnel trained to train the foodaholic how to develop the proper THINKING about diet and lifestyle.

2) More important, without realizing it, Weight Watchers is constantly reminding one that he is fat—the major mistake of almost all weight programs except mine, and a few others. I'll go into great detail on this soon.

LET YOURSELF
RATIONALIZE NO FURTHER!

You are, in all probability, a foodaholic. But you must admit same before any significant change can be accomplished. NOW is the time to cease your flimsy excuses—your complex rationalizations. Now is the time to admit your chronic need to obsessively-compulsively eat. NOW is the time to begin a re-newed lifestyle. Now is the time to be "born again" into the world of the slender, energetic people. Now!

FINAL NOTE

The type of diet you may pursue on my program is not important at this time. Neither is the type of exercise program. These will both naturally take care of themselves "magically" as you soon watch the step-by-step development of my program in Part II. All you need do at this point is to flat-out admit to yourself that you ARE a foodaholic and discontinue NOW making any more excuses for it and/or rationalizing your indulgent behavior.

CHAPTER THREE

*Probable
Causes of Foodaholism*

OBSESSIVE-COMPULSIVE EATING

We have already established that you are, in all probability a foodaholic, an obsessive-compulsive eater. Obsessive-compulsive means just what it says: Freud first called it a psychic fixation, it is the "MUST" performance of a ritual or behavior pattern. A "COMMAND PERFORMANCE;" an "OFFER WE CAN'T REFUSE;" something we know we should not do, but we can't help ourselves; a craving that we fulfill to spite, and in spite of, ourselves.

· It is classified in psychology as a neurosis, especially if the ritual is any manner destructive to self or others—which most obsession-compulsions are. There would be very few types of behavior one could list (lying, stealing, gambling, drinking, sexual, etc.) that at least someone does not have a fixation or "HANG-UP" towards. But in our case in this book we will deal with the overwhelming "HUNGER" for food.

CAUSAL FACTORS

There are many theories as to the origin of obsessive-compulsive eating and there is ample research to give at least some validity to all of them. One of the following may well be the reason you are a foodaholic—and there is a distinct possibility (even probability) that it is a combination of all of the following. They are NOT written in any special order of importance.

A) ORAL FIXATION

Sigmund Freud very astutely, and correctly, first pointed out that we humans (and select other higher animals) go through a period from birth to approximately 1-1/2 years old in which our entire psychic energy, our entire being is focused in on our mouth. We instinctively know that our mouth and its relationship to our mother's breast or breast substitute, is our entire survival. Not only do we get our milk, water, and food from the source of our survival (mother, mom, momma) through the mouth, but Freud also first noted that the mouth is surrounded by sensitive membrane that, when stimulated, reduces tension and stress. By the way, it is interesting to note that all the other direct openings of the human body are also surrounded by sensitive tissue, that, when stimulated, also reduce tension and stress and give pleasure, but that's another topic for another book.

In any event, ALL of us "LEARN" early that eating or sticking almost anything in our mouth to either suck or chew, brings us much pleasure and reduces or eliminates pain—the entire nature of Freud's "ID". However, it is also obvious that some humans not only "LEARN" this pattern, but learn it extremely strong. They not only like to stimulate their oral region, they LOVE it, crave it, become obsessed with it, and are compulsed (self-forced) to do it. They develop this pattern very early in life and most will carry, and even further develop, this pattern the remainder of their lives. This phenomenon is characterized as a psychic fixation at the oral stage—more commonly known as an oral fixation.

If oral fixators do not have a breast to stick in their mouth, no problem! They simply discover that the world is chock full of breast substitutes—nipples, pacifiers, thumbs, food substances, pencils, ice chewing, security blankets, nailbiting, cigarettes, chewing gum, chewing tobacco, pipes, snuff, ad infinitum. You name it, they shove it in their mouth simply for the temporary stimulation and stress relief it provides.

By the way, I never cease to be amazed how often habitual tobacco users try to deny the above to themselves and others. Actually, tobacco is a very low addiction drug which produces very few withdrawal symptoms when withdrawn. It is the psychological addiction (oral fixation) which has the person "HOOKED" and this is the major reason most people claim to gain weight when they stop smoking. Of course most do, because they substitute food substance for the tobacco, just as they at one time substituted tobacco for the breast.

Also, our tobacco usage is sad commentary as to how weirdly we humans have developed our rituals. If I sit at a banquet—or in a bar—with a woman's breast in my mouth, I'll go to jail or a mental institution. If I sit there with my thumb in my mouth, people will laugh at me, lose respect for me, and call me babified. But if I substitute a cigarette or pipe, I am suave and sophisticated. Yet, the pipe or cigarette is the only one of the three above that is destructive to me and others around me. Whew!

Back to the point. Why do some people develop this highly exaggerated oral fixation and some don't, even though they have similar early experiences. We flat-out don't know—yet! That would be like asking me why four people riding in one car to work hear three songs on the radio. One person has one of the songs fixated (running through his head) the remainder of the day; person #2 has another, person #3 another, and person #4 none of the three. There are simply too many variables within the 10 billion thinking cells in the cerebral cortex to know the "WHY'S", at least at this time. But, most important for now, we DO know that these fixations take place and that they are very destructive, degrading, and debilitating to us.

In all probability, those people who do begin to develop such fixations early do so due to two exaggerated relationships with their mother, and possibly to a lesser degree with their father: 1) an over-indulging relationship in which they are "SMOTHER-LOVED" incessantly. That is, they are constantly getting a breast of some kind to stick in their mouth and they are learning strongly that succorance and biting is simply the way life is. They need something (or someone) to suck on or bite on. They know nothing else.

2) The opposite: Mother or parental deprivation. Either they were deprived of the breast, which represents both food and love/affection or they at least interpreted their life so. Therefore, they start developing a pattern of "I DON'T HAVE ENOUGH BREAST (FOOD, AFFECTION). I NEED IT, PLEASE GIVE ME SOME, PLEASE MOMMY, PLEASE, PLEASE, PLEASE!"

They are "STARVED" (interesting slang term, isn't it?) for affection; feel deprived; and thus spend the rest of their lives (usually) sticking breasts and breast substitutes in their mouths. You see, when the old Jewish Bible writers said, "BRING A CHILD UP IN THE WAY HE SHOULD GO AND HE'LL NEVER PART FROM IT" they probably didn't even realize just HOW correct they were. And, of course, if they were right, then the inverse is true: "BRING A CHILD UP IN THE WAY HE SHOULDN'T GO, AND HE'LL NEVER PART FROM THAT EITHER." But, as I'll show you, the only wrong word in the above two quotes is NEVER. Any person can change.

I must tell you, at this point, that there is no question in my mind that my own father, a severe foodaholic, was a product of this deprivation syndrome. I saw it surface during his entire life, both physiologically ("I NEED FOOD, BADLY!") and psychologically ("I NEED LOVE AND ATTENTION, BADLY!"). He carried it to his death-bed. "Eleanor (my mother) give me food, please give me food, please give me food, I'm hungry," he begged and pleaded until he died. It was a tragic scene from a man I loved. It was quite natural that he selected (fell in love with) a highly nurturant woman who, though she didn't realize it, loved to stick her breast (food) in his mouth; thrived on nurturing her man—and children—and needed his succorance and dependance upon her. This is a very common pattern among deprivation men (and nurturant women). And, unfortunately, there are always many highly nurturant people—mommies, daddies, nurses, grandma's, restaurant cooks, etc.—ready, willing and able to show their "LOVE" by sticking a breast in the foodaholics mouth. It's exactly like waiting around the street corner to find a wino so that you can pour wine down his throat and then saying, "Well, he should be able to keep his mouth shut and not let me do that!"

B) FOOD AS
A REWARD—PUNISHMENT SYSTEM

There is another well-accepted theory about obsessive-compulsive eating that I believe also has merit. Let's discuss it briefly. Parents, particularly mothers, (leave it to me to always attack flag, apple pie, Chevrolets and motherhood) unwittingly develop food—our most needed life source—as a very complex, sophisticated punishment-reward system within their children. I could give thousands of examples of how they "TRANSACT" this without realizing it; but following are choice ones:

1) "If you're good, I'll bake some cookies later."

2) "If you don't quit that, you'll get sent to bed without supper."

3) "If you'll carry out the trash, we'll get an ice cream cone downtown."

4) "You were bad, you don't get any candy."

5) Etc., etc., etc.

Unconsciously, living with this system day after day, week after week, month after month, year after year, the child internalizes this deadly pattern. That is, the food punishment-reward system becomes a part of his very deepest being and he begins to treat himself in the same manner as his parents treated him. For example, when he feels he has done something good (say a job promotion), he then rewards himself ("Honey, let's go out to celebrate"—which usually means "pigging out" at a fancy restaurant).

Even worse, when he (she) feels "bad"—that is uptight, tense and stressful—he tries to feel "good" by rewarding himself with food. Little wonder that almost all you foodaholics will tell me that the more uptight and pressured you feel, the more you head for the refrigerator and pantry ("Honey, whatever you got, get it out"). This, along with oral fixations, also explains why you will continue to stuff yourself even after you no longer are really hungry. Sound familiar? Don't you often almost need a ramrod to keep getting those peanuts or potato chips down far after hunger pangs are gone? I've been down that road many times?

There is also widespread foodaholism within my mother's side of the family and I am convinced that most of it stems from a combination of the overindulgent oral fixation syndrome discussed earlier and the reward-punishment system above. My Grandfather Henry personified both—as did my Grandmother. Coincidentally or maybe not so coincidentally, his entire life was built around, and dedicated to, the grocery (food) business.

OBESITY IN CHILDREN

While on this topic, I wish to make a strong statement on gross obesity in children since this seems to be the appropriate place. There is absoutely no excuse, other than rare organic causes, for excessive fatness in children. My eyes moisten almost every time I observe a "fat kid" because I know the life style he has already strongly begun; where it is surely bound to lead him; and the hardships and heartaches he'll endure along the way.

Parents (mainly mother, again) do their children a great disservice when they fatten them like forced-fed calves. And, sadly, they usually do so in the name of love ("It shows my family love when I cook big meals all the time" and "It shows love for me and my cooking when they ask for second and third helpings of my wonderful cooking") and health ("A fat child with fat cheeks and thighs and fat little belly is a healthy child.")

Sorry, Charlie—and Charletta,—a fat child is only that, a FAT child. And you have him well on his way to further fatness, poor self-concept, open-heart surgery at 45, high blood pressure, stroke, depression, guilt, etc. Proud of yourself, Mommy? The over-feeding of sugars, starches, and fats to a child is parallel in the long run to permitting him to be run over by a drunk driver. Where are our M.A.D.D. Mothers when we need them? (See next chapter).

C) HEREDITY AND CELLULAR PRE-DISPOSITION

As you may realize, there is a great deal of research being conducted presently regarding the feasibility of ALCOHOLISM being hereditary. Many scientists and psychologists believe that some people inherit a pre-disposition to cellular make-up that craves or can't tolerate alcohol. IF this is proven true, which in my opinion very possibly will be but hasn't yet, then a person will be able to take a test at birth or early infancy, and determine immediately whether or not he is destined to be alcoholic.

Well, there is also a school of thought (not widely developed) that the same may be true of foodaholism. Could it be true that there is also a tendency proneness or pre-disposition to inherited cellular make-up that "craves" food substances. I, personally, do not think so, but as a rational thinker, must leave open his possibility—though it hasn't yet been proven.

It is true, no question, that we do inherit body types that convert food substances almost immediately to adipose tissue or types that do NOT readily do so. Don't we "easy-converters" detest and despise the "hard-converters?"—those who can eat all they please and never become obese? Wouldn't it be pure heaven to possess such a body-type? The universial laws ("God") played a cruel trick on us.

It is also theorized that we seem to almost have a pre-disposed "target" weight that our minds and bodies work toward, gravitate to, and relentlessly strive for. Again, however, I put little stock in this or hereditary cellular disposition. And even IF it is all true, I do know beyond a shadow of a doubt that the target weight can be altered; that foodaholism can be "whooped"; that cellular pre-disposition can be conquered; and that weight can be lost and kept off. I have done it! I have helped hundreds of others do it. My success rate is 90%—compared to the national average of 5% and up to 15% with most other programs. That's right, you read correctly—90%! And I can even pick out my unsuccessful 10% candidates quickly so as not to waste their time and/or money—and my time. Furthermore, it is not as difficult as you may think. And it is fun—if you follow my principles. THERE ARE NO LEGITIMATE EXCUSES FOR BEING FAT—ONLY EXCUSES!

D) GUILT (SHAME)

Seven years ago, I published a book titled **GUILT—GO TO HELL!** Even with no marketing except my own and word-of-mouth, the book has sold well over 30,000 copies and I have hundreds of letters on file from people stating that the book strengthened the quality of their lives or changed their lives entirely. The book is out of print now, though I plan a revised re-write soon. In any event, the royalties I garnered from that book were ALL given to charity. The rewards gathered from readers were quite sufficient for me at that time.

However, the point is that the entire book deals with the ranges of guilt and how to overcome this terrible emotion. It is the most destructive, degrading, and debilitating of all the human emotions and it eats people up and spits them out alive! When one mentions guilt, most people usually put it in a religious context, but religious guilt is only a small part of this awesome emotion. To a psychologist, guilt is any form of the following:

F.O.P.B.A.F.B.Y.D.M.C.S.S.

FEAR OF PUNISHMENT BY AUTHORITY FIGURES BECAUSE YOU DON'T MEET CERTAIN SET STANDARDS!

There are literally thousands of ways in which "guilt trips" (a great term coined by our youth) are laid on us constantly. Some people, tragically, so internalize this "I don't measure up" syndrome that their self-concept, self-image, identity, ego-strength—whatever term you wish to use—becomes shattered. Sometimes this happens early in life, sometimes it takes longer to "break" a person's self-esteem. But it's only a matter of time.

And whenever it eventually occurs, it becomes quite common for that person to turn to food in order to "prove" (usually unconsciously) to himself just how unworthy, shameful, and despicable he is. He literally "gives up and gives in" and sets on a steady course toward suicide by food. He hasn't the nerve to put a gun to his head or jump off a bridge so he simply does it through knife, fork, and spoon. This person almost always scores high on depression scales (guilt scales) when taking a personality test.

This was another pattern which described and characterized my own father for most of his life. It was also my own pattern for the majority of my prime years on this earth. You who have not experienced it can never fathom it's "fire and rain" upon your existence!

E) HEREDITY OF EATING HABITS

Are you serious? It is morbid how often I have heard my clients (and others) state: "I'm this way because I inherited my fatness and eating habits from one (or both) of my parents and grandparents." What a pure, hybrid copout this is! While it may possibly be true that we inherit a body, molecular, cellular, and metabolic make-up that easily converts sugars and starches into fat, to rationalize obesity as a hereditary problem is pure "gobbledygook!" I might accept emotional disturbance, emotional upheaval, depression or environmental eating patterns of some type—but don't lay the HEREDITY defecation on me. Spare me, please! I get my intelligence insulted enough—and so do you.

F) "SLENDERAPHOBIA"

Let's really get into some deep psychology for a moment. But I promise to keep the wording and concepts simple. There is no question in my mind—based on my experience, research and reading—that a good many grossly overweight people suffer from what I choose to call "SLENDERAPHOBIA." That is, they actually have an exaggerated fear of LOSING their fat. I have seen this first-hand on many occasions and it is witnessed by the fact that so many chronically obese people will make statements such as "Why, I might get down to nothing" or "Well, I'm afraid if I get too carried away with this weight loss thing, I might develop anorexia." At first, it will seem they are saying all this in jest but as you get to know them in counseling sessions, you soon learn that they are dead serious.

Sigmund Freud originated the theory of Feces Retention. Though Feces Retention is too lengthy and deep to be discussed here, suffice it to say that a) it is well-accepted by many psychologists today; b) I certainly see clearly how this lifelong pattern of "keeping what is mine to myself" manifests itself in some people; and c) I believe Feces Retention to be the basis of some chronic obesity—and most certainly, "SLENDERAPHOBIA."

In simple terms, we know that many people have early developed fixations (hang-ups) regarding strict hesitation to part with ANYTHING that is a part of them—yes, even their defecation! Children with this condition will literally withhold their bowel movement until either going in their pants or getting sick. It was Freud's belief that a) this was a form of resentment against a rigid, yet distant parent; and b) that it later in life carried over to a highly-conservative retention of other personal values—such as money. (That's where the term "tightwad" originated. Most Feces Retainers will develop a tightwad.)

Well, I'm convinced that there is a significant percentage of people who have retained their fat for so long that they have a deep fear of giving it up. Hence, "SLENDERAPHOBIA."

G) DEPRESSION

Functional depression and organic depression (physical/chemical causes) also seem to lead many people to eat incessantly. They usually claim that the pleasures of food are their "only joys of life." Functional depression is a direct product of guilt—which I've already explained. It is simply aggression turned in on self. And since obesity almost always causes further guilt and poor self-concept, overeating eventually only makes the depression worsen. So again, the foodaholic is entrapped and enmeshed in a vicious cycle.

It should be added here that it has been my experience through the years that RARELY does a grossly overweight person have a truly wholesome self-concept. I've had many of my obese counselees and students attempt to convince me that they do but they are usually trying harder to convince themselves than me. I have offered them the opportunity to look at a picture of themselves through a pupillametrics device. If they're correct about their over-all good self-image, the pupils of their eyes should dilate upon viewing their picture. I'm willing to bet them a steak dinner their pupils contract. THAT'S THE NAME OF THAT TUNE!

H) APPROACH-AVOIDANCE CONFLICT AND POOR COPING STRATEGIES

You may be aware of an old term used in the field of psychology—approach-avoidance conflict. If not, it simply means that as we humans encounter life's daily problems and transactions, we constantly must make decisions regarding whether to confront and solve these little (or big) vicissitudes or to run away from these hardships and "hide" in some manner. A kind of "Make the world go away" syndrome.

I have found that many foodaholics and "junk food junkies" are persons who are largely avoidance personalities. And for whatever reason, food and obesity becomes their form of hiding. In other words, they have developed POOR COPING STRATEGIES in the daily tasks of living. Naturally, to coin an old cliche, they can't run away from their problems—at least, not in the vast majority of cases. But they still attempt to do so, and food and fat is the vehicle they have chosen for their "getaway car." Of course, that car breaks down—both physically and psychologically/emotionally—and they are stranded on the highway of life. One might also call it "being up the creek without a spoon." Almost without exception, those people eat themselves to death VERY PREMATURELY unless they diligently pursue a program like mine. Their problems run deep!

I) COGNITIVE DISTURBANCE

You probably are not aware of a counseling approach used by some therapists called COGNITIVE THERAPY. One of the major premises of said approach is that you must learn to let your thoughts affect your emotional moods rather than permit your moods to control your thoughts—as most people quite often do. The key words in cognitive therapy are "thought control" and the counselor's expertise is in teaching his client the techniques for doing so.

A large percentage of obsessive-compulsive eaters suffer a serious disturbance in their cognitive balance. That is to say, their moods so dictate their daily conception and interpretation of life that they sort of live a life of confusion. Therefore, food seems to become their only contact with stability. That is why they usually "head for the refrigerator" when any negative event occurs in their life. It is my experience that those who suffer this problem are usually also very rigid, regimented people in their moral beliefs. For this reason, they are difficult clients and though they very much need to read and digest a book such as this one, they usually won't even complete reading it. They'll find something in it to "conveniently" offend them. If you happen to recognize yourself as possibly fitting this profile, do yourself one of the greatest favors of your life and DON'T LAY THIS BOOK DOWN! Even if you are offended by some of my words or phrasing.

J) INHERITED TARGET WEIGHT?

Just recently, after almost completing the entire manuscript for this book, I saw a TV show (on national network, mind you) which took the strong stance that a human being inherits at birth a pre-disposed target weight and that he is, therefore, pre-destined to be fat no matter what he does. The show was entitled "America's Obsession with Thin" or something to that effect and it was the darndest bunch of gobbledygook I've ever seen.

The show spent an hour quoting a few so-called "experts" who defended the above research. But the main messages of the show were "Accept being fat;" "Learn to live with it;" "You can't change it, no matter what you do;" "Forget trying to become slender, there is no way;" and "Fat is fine."

I could not believe that I was viewing this on national TV—realizing that so many people believe anything they see on TV and accept it as gospel. You see, when P. T. Barnum allegedly stated "There is a fool born every minute," he was dead wrong. There is far more than one "fool" born every minute.

In any event, there is absolutely no doubt in my mind that large food corporations financially backed the making of that "documentary." And if they didn't, they sure were happy to see it. Well, it's pure bull_____! As I have mentioned previously, while it is quite obvious that we do inherit body types, metabolic tendencies, etc., we do not inherit target weights. And even if we did (or do), to say that that target weight can't be altered downward and maintained thusly is simply not true. I, and many, many others, have proved that it is done—and quite easily, thank you! I'll show you how.

CHAPTER FOUR

The Origination of M.A.F.I.A.

This book will also serve as the beginning "kick-off" of a group I am forming called M.A.F.I.A.—MOTHERS AGAINST FAT IN AMERICA!

It is altogether fitting and proper that this national movement bear the name M.A.F.I.A. Just as the Sicilian Cosa Nostra we call Mafia swept into America and became an awesome power movement which preyed on the "grass roots" person in this country—slowly but surely destructing not only each person, but ravenously devouring the very innards of society with its greed, corruption, and deceit, SO DOES FAT!

As already noted, no health problem in America—including cancer, alcohol, and drugs—even comes close to obesity in the destructiveness it wroughts. Foodaholism and our obsession with grease, refined sugar, cholesterol and huge quantities of carbohydrates in this country is the major reason millions of Americans die prematurely due to heart attacks, sugar diabetes, strokes, stemming from hypertension, etc. It is also the chief cause of senility, arteriosclerosis, and possibly Alzheimer's disease.

The giant corporate conglomerates dealing with "destructive" food substances have sold us a bill of goods on a magnanimous level through their mass media advertising campaigns. They literally have us eating ourselves to death and enjoying it. It reminds me of the humorous definition of tact: "Being able to tell a person to go to hell and have him glad to be on his way!"

These giant corporations are no better than the underworld Mafia, and very possibly many of them are controlled by the Mafia now that their vast amounts of money from gambling, cocaine, heroin, prostitution, etc. are being "laundered" into "legitimate" business. The "common-herd" person in this country simply has no concept of how much money, power, and devastation is involved—just as most of you had never stopped to think how much your diet is controlled by these big food interests and their commercials—including their take-over of Saturday morning TV time so as to "brainwash" your children to PROPER (ha! ha!) eating habits. They condition us from womb to tomb!! Almost all their beautifully conceived advertisements have the same theme: "Eat, eat, eat" and "Eat yourself to death!"

And that brings us back to M.A.F.I.A.—MOTHERS AGAINST FAT IN AMERICA. Many of you probably think I'm not serious or that I'm writing "tongue in cheek" on this issue. REST ASSURED THAT I AM DEAD SERIOUS about the creation of this group and I will now detail why—along with the purposes and goals of M.A.F.I.A.

1) LET'S GET MAD!

We presently have a group in America called M.A.D.D.—Mothers Against Drunk Drivers. They are raising a lot of cane, and rightfully so, about the death and destruction wrought on our highways by drunken drivers. A group called S.A.D.D.—Students Against Drunk Drivers—has joined them, as have many law enforcement officials and judges, both of whom have traditionally jumped on any bandwagon which would give them more power. And the drunken driver crackdown is a great power instrument because no one in his right mind can be against it. I strongly support it also, though I'm cautious as to the implications of how it might be enforced, over-enforced or enforced with inequity. Nevertheless, who can argue against getting drunks off the highway?

WELL, WOMEN OF M.A.D.D., I WOULD LIKE TO STRONGLY RE-MIND YOU THAT ALCOHOL DOESN'T EVEN COME CLOSE TO DE-STROYING AS MANY OF YOUR YOUNG CHILDREN—BOTH PHYSI-CALLY AND EMOTIONALLY—AS DOES OBESITY AND PRESENT AMERICAN DIETARY HABITS, NOT EVEN CLOSE!

But because it happens in a different manner (less violent) and usually has a slower onset (though not always), you hadn't thought of it that way, had you? If a significant amount of mothers are getting "bent out of shape" regarding drunken drivers, then we should have fantastic amounts of mothers up in arms and "raising cane about sugar cane," grease, fat, cholesterol, etc.

Instead, most of you not only had not thought of it—you promote it. In the name of love—and in the name of ignorance—you think that fattening up your kid (by the way, for the "slaughter"—that is, the heart surgeon some day) is a sign of good, loving, caring motherhood. Little do you know that you are simply teaching him early patterns which will soon lead him to obesity, poor health, poor self-concept, depression, withdrawal, etc. for the remainder of his life. Due to emotional problems, guilt and shame, a very small percentage of overeaters never regain their full potentials and creativity—and even those who do are either too obese to REALLY, TRULY enjoy their success or their health is gone prematurely anyway. And I really shouldn't have to tell you that even conquering the world is only a shallow, hollow, empty victory if your health is gone, anyway.

I want to relate to you a scene I witnessed just yesterday, but it is a scenario I've seen thousands of times in my lifetime: a friend of mine owns a nice restaurant in this area and his wife works with him as one of the cooks. Their son (probably about 10 years old) is already extremely obese. You'll soon see why.

The boy was sitting in the bar/lounge area with me and had just come home from school. It was approximately 4:30 p.m. and he was watching TV. His mother asked him if he was hungry. He, of course, replied in the affirmative. The bar had many baskets of potato chips, cornchips, taco chips and pretzels for patrons to munch. While engrossed in an episode of Bugs Bunny, he had already devoured one entire basket of cornchips. His mother soon brought in a large hamburger, a large order of french fries and a large cola. The boy drank the cola quickly and she brought him another.

He "wolfed down" (literally) this meal quickly and started on a basket of potato chips. About this time, the bartenderess brought in a vegetable plate with dip and a cheese ball with an assortment of crackers. I found myself at least hoping he'd "hit" the vegetable plate—but he went straight for the crackers and cheese, even dipping them into the dip. I was getting full—and even sick—just watching him. He'd probably already inhaled over 2,000 calories worth of at best what would be considered low-nutrition food.

Soon Bugs Bunny gave way to the Flintstones. Mother re-appeared and asked him if he was still hungry? He said yes (and I darn near fell off my stool). Since I know this family, I tried to jokingly say, "I don't see how on earth he could be hungry." She laughed and commented, "Oh, Jerry, he's still a growing boy and he loves mom's cooking, don't you, honey?" The boy nodded affirmative in no uncertain terms and ate some pretzels until his "loving" mom returned with ANOTHER large hamburger, ANOTHER larger order of fries and a milkshake!

My thoughts at that moment: "Woman, you know not what havoc you are wreaking on this young child—a minor." If she were giving him pot they would charge her with contributing to the delinquency of a minor. The rejection and teasing he'll probably encounter; the burdensome life patterns he'll endure all his life; the health problems he'll soon have (10 years, 20 years, 30 years, it will come quickly because life is like a breeze passing over a field of wheat); the rationalizations he'll soon have to develop—both to himself and others—to "save face" for his foodaholism; the lack of self-concept and pride in appearance he'll feel, etc., ad infinitum. I know. I've been there. "If I were king of the world—which I'm not and don't wish to be—mothers like her wouldn't even be allowed to have children. I know, I know, it's a free country, right? But keep in mind that if she abused him physically, we would take him away from her. Well, I contend she IS abusing him physically!

My further thoughts: "Let's say that 500 (more or less?) children are actually killed by drunken drivers each year in the U. S. I'll bet my very life that more children—even under 12—actually die each year in America due to extreme obesity, fat around the heart, etc. But even IF I'm wrong, I do know that these children are quickly and surely being "killed" indirectly. HELL WOMEN, YOU'D BE BETTER OFF QUITTING M.A.D.D., JOINING THE M.A.F.I.A. AND TAKING YOUR CHANCES WITH THE DRUNKS! Better still, join both! If you don't want drunks taking potshots at him on the highways, then why don't you refrain from developing his "pot gut" in the kitchenways?

2) JOIN US CHILD ABUSE OPPONENTS

The good mothers of our country are also very upset about child abuse—as are you and I—and again, rightfully so. Being abused is so utterly devastating to a young child and usually affects the remainder of his life in a negative manner, right? Yes, we have conclusive documentation of same. It is well-established that most assaultive adults have been severely abused either emotionally and/or physically as children.

Well, once again, child abuse does not even touch childhood obesity as a major problem in this country. And the overall effects of childhood—and therefore, life-long—foodaholism are just as debilitating, as already discussed. But since foodaholism isn't as dramatic and therefore not as newsworthy to the media, most of you hadn't thought of it, had you?

In fact, it is my contention that "force feeding" and "feeder'calfing" children, as so many mothers and grandmothers do, DOES CONSTITUTE CHILD ABUSE! I mean that mothers of America! Hate me? You are causing eventual emotional and physical scar tissue that is almost as bad as "slapping them up the side of the head." So, wonderful women, if you are going to crusade against child abuse, fine. But join the M.A.F.I.A., too, won't you?

3) C'MON NANCY

Just this week, Nancy Reagan, our First Lady, convened first ladies of the nation and world in a joint effort to protect our children from drug abuse. This is a worthy cause and worthwhile movement, Mrs. Reagan, and I applaud you. I was once a director of a drug and alcohol abuse program and I know first hand that drug abuse is most surely a "LONG, LONELY ROAD TO NOWHERE!" However, Mrs. Reagan, you guessed it. Drug abuse as a western world social problem does not even approach food abuse! Not one iota! But since many large food processing corporate conglomerates probably support your husband (as do I), it would be most difficult for you to convene a blue ribbon group of first ladies on food abuse, obesity and poor dietary habits in our children, wouldn't it? You see, all those companies, and many others like them, love it when we "ramrod" as much of their junk food as possible down our throats—or the throats of our children. Their stockholders thrive on it and their survival depends upon it. Can you imagine the American Restaurant Association introducing a food education program? That would be like asking stripminers to introduce land reclamation; or politicians to vote themselves pay cuts; or drunks to initiate M.A.D.D.; or to leave your dog to guard the meat market. But women, if you're against the ravages of drug abuse in our children, you must be against the less dramatic—but more degrading—food abuse epidemic which plagues our country. Join M.A.F.I.A.!

4) "WELL, IT'S A FREE COUNTRY, AFTER ALL!"

At this point, probably many of you reading this are making the above statement. And, of course, the answer is obviously a resounding "YES!" There is no one who believes in personal, individual liberties more than Jerry Walke. I've even often wondered why we do not have a national holiday for Thomas Jefferson—in my mind the greatest human being who ever lived because he, more than any other person, was able to detail and put into words what it means for a human being to be free to live and roam in the universe. And the average "grass roots" person does not comprehend how essential the American Civil Liberties Union is to our way of life.

Certainly one can eat himself/herself to death if he/she wishes. Or drink himself to death. Or drug himself to death. Or jump off a bridge. Had it occurred to you that the greatest freedom one has in a free country is to commit suicide? Or dress as he wishes. Or worship, speak, write or believe whatever he desires. But we have laws so that one cannot force these rights on others and therefore do damage to them. That's what M.A.D.D. and S.A.D.D. are all about, and child abuse laws, and drug laws. And though I'm not stupid enough to believe it will happen in the near future, we do need laws to protect CHILDREN from food abuse by adults. I truly believe that! But the nation is not ready—at least not yet—for the laws to govern this commonly practiced, SOCIALLY-ACCEPTABLE abuse of the child. Therefore, M.A.F.I.A. will concern itself, for the time being, with educational programs and news media commercials to educate our population. Education has always been far more effective than attempting to legislate morality, anyway.

5) ATTENTION:
KENNY ROGERS, LIONEL RITCHIE
AND MICHAEL JACKSON!

Do you have any choice but to join M.A.F.I.A.? You recently organized a beautiful tape session with many of the leading entertainers in the world to help the starving hordes of Africa. God Bless You! It was so well done and the music/singing were most impressive. I have donated and, in fact, help sponsor an Ethiopian child. You cannot be praised enough for your efforts.

But, as mentioned earlier, look at the irony of it all. Our children in America running around with bellies bloated with food while theirs are bloated with the water of starvation—our children with layers of fat on their ribs while their ribs stick out. Throw your weight and influence behind M.A.F.I.A. and help us to educate our young mothers and young children. Our young women do not need to think that love means continually sticking their breasts (and later, the breast substitutes—spoons and forks) into their childrens' mouths. Let us begin to teach together!

6) GOALS

The major thrust and only true goal of M.A.F.I.A.—at this time—will be to enlighten our people regarding the physical and emotional suffering of food abuse and to educate them (as this book does) to proper psychological and physical approaches to food.

We will accomplish this through mass media, by mail, and by word-of-mouth. We will not only inform Americans of proper dietary habits, but use self-concept psychology to appeal to their sense of pride, humanitarianism, development of potential and development of creativity.

We need to use our "clout" to become guests on TV shows such as Johnny Carson and Phil Donahue. We need to tell our story on prime time TV and radio. Rest assured that our "opposition" does so.

7) HOW ABOUT CRITICS?

If we influence just one parent not to destroy her/his child by internalizing within him this burden of foodaholism at a young age, then it will be worth all the criticism that I'm certain the obese people and food corporations of this country will heap upon us. In fact, their attacks on us will probably constitute a defense mechanism (cover-up), rationalization of their own foodaholism anyway. "If the shoe (or any other article of clothing) fits, let them wear it!"

Sure, I'm being tough again. But M.A.D.D. and S.A.D.D. are tough. And child abuse groups are tough. And law enforcement folks are tough. It is time for parents to refrain and abstain from pushing their "fat-catness" onto their offspring. Our critics? "Let them eat cake."

To close this section on the origination of M.A.F.I.A., below is a letter I sent to *60 Minutes* following a segment they did on a group attempting to remove beer commercials from TV:

May 6, 1985

Morley Safer
60 Minutes
CBS
51 West 52nd Street
New York, New York 10019

Dear Morley:

Any knowledgeable doctor will tell you that food abuse is by far our most destructive health problem in America today—including youth. Censor Budwiser and Miller Lite commercials today, McDonald's and Wendy's tomorrow.

I guess I'll form M.A.F.I.A.—Mothers Against Fat In America!

Sincerely,

Dr. Jerry L. Walke
Portsmouth, Ohio 45662

It should be noted that I, as a great believer in the free enterprise system and freedom itself, do not wish to censor any food commercial. I was even against censoring liquor and tobacco commercials. But I do believe that M.A.F.I.A. should be formed to tell the other side of the story to the public. And, most certainly, if tobacco ads must be accompanied by a "smoking may be hazardous to your health" statement, then so equally should all ads selling refined sugar, grease, cholesterol, etc. Any rational thinking, "common sense" person should agree.

CHAPTER FIVE

Research On Obesity

INTRODUCTION . . .

We have conducted a great deal of research on obese people. It is very SENSITIVE research since I realize that there are organizations representing obese people (why don't we just say "fat"?) and because I've been an obese person most of my life and because foodaholism is so prevalent in my family. But, let it be known that we've conducted all the following research as fairly, genuinely and scientifically as possible—that is, trying to allow for as many variables as we possibly could. Every attempt has been made to allow for reliability (consistency) and validity. We've diligently tried not to "weight" our samplings, keeping them as random as possible. We've strived hard not to bias or halo our work.

Angee Whitt, a non-foodaholic and a registered nurse with "no axes to grind," aided me in putting together the research. In particular, she both snapped and assembled the various photograph series which we'll be discussing. Her presence further insured the non-bias that we wanted to achieve. It may well be that some of the results will be offensive to some of you, but we are simply reporting what we found.

BEAUTY
PREFERENCE AND DISCRIMINATION

It is quite obvious that there is an emphasis placed on beauty in all of mankind and especially in western civilization. This is easily "proved" in America alone by the simple fact that most of us don't mind eating beef of some kind yet will balk (especially women) at eating deer meat. Why? simply because the deer is more beautiful than the cow. There are all types of research to show that, in many areas of society, attractive women gain preferential treatment over not-so-attractive women; that good-looking men gain ample advantages over not-so-good-looking men; and that well-dressed people attain all kinds of one-ups-manship over not-so-well dressed persons. It's simply a fact of life that so many crucial decisions ranging from political voting to job securement and from mate selection to court decisions are made based upon physical appearances. That is simply a fact of life! Therefore, we set out in our research to discover how much (or how little) grossly overweight people suffer from discrimination, negative bias, and non-preferential treatment.

I personally interviewed the president or director of personnel of 100 small manufacturing companies in Ohio, Kentucky and West Virginia. They were promised complete anonymity because many seemed to fear some form of discrimination charge—though I'm not sure exactly what that charge could be under current law.

I first asked an overt question with no conditions, "Do you hire any grossly overweight persons in your company?" (I defined grossly overweight as I do throughout this book—anyone who is 30 lbs. or more above what they should reasonably weigh for their body frame and stature.) Nine of the 100 answered flatly "No!" Seven answered "Yes" and 84 responded "sometimes," "at times," or something similar.

I then asked those nine, "Why?" Three answered for health reasons. One answered for health and image of the company reasons. Two responded "image of the company" only. Three said it was because lack of discipline in eating is usually indicative of lack of discipline in other areas essential to company success.

I then asked the other 91 executives a second question. "You have two applicants for the same position. They are of the same sex, race, religion, etc. and have exactly the same qualifications in terms of training, credentials, references and interviewing skills. The ONLY difference is that one is slim and trim and the other is grossly overweight. Which would you hire? Are you ready? Eighty-seven of the 91 stated that they would hire the slim and trim one. Two said they'd flip a coin. Two said they'd hire the grossly overweight. ALL FOUR EXECUTIVES WHO DID NOT RESPOND "SLIM AND TRIM" WERE THEMSELVES GROSSLY OVERWEIGHT!

Based on this elementary little piece of research, one might conclude that if you are obese and job-hunting, you might be wise to begin by selecting an obese employer. But it certainly was obvious, at least in this small but significant sampling, that companies prefer to employ slender persons over obese ones.

RESPECT RESEARCH

Over the past six years, I've conducted a longitudinal piece of research that is very interesting to me. I will not attest to its validity or reliability. Neither am I certain that I've taken into account all variables. Therefore, I don't present it to you as SCIENTIFIC research, but I think you'll agree its statistical implications are worth pondering.

In my classes within a community college setting, I get many adults—both male and female—returning for additional educational training. Anytime I have an older person in my class, I make a point sometime during the quarter of calling that person aside privately and asking him/her if he has children. IF the answer is affirmative, I then ask if he/she would be willing to place the over-all respect they get from their children on a scale from zero (no respect) to five (excellent respect)—one representing very little; two indicating below average; three meaning average; and four equaling quite good. Most of these adult students have participated in my little study.

Without their knowledge, I note whether that parent is slender, somewhat obese or grossly overweight. Of course, I later record this—plus the sex of the parent and the numerical score they give themselves.

Over the years, I've compiled a great sampling—753 mothers and 612 fathers to be exact. And I believe the computerized statistics are somewhat relevant. The mean (average) score for slender mothers was 4.2 and for slender fathers 4.1. The mean score for somewhat obese mothers was 3.6 and for somewhat obese fathers 3.4. The average score for grossly overweight mothers was 3.2 and for the same type father ONLY 2.8! Realizing the limitations of this "informal" research, there still seems to me to be some messages about obesity and the respect factor. Epecially since the sampling was large AND the participants rated themselves. In my opinion, the implications of the above scores are multifaceted—and staggering! Obese parents, by their own evaluations, did not believe that they were getting nearly as much respect from their children as did slender parents. Quite frankly, over-all they were probably correct. I'll discuss why in my self-concept chapters.

SIDEWALK CONSTRUCTION SITE

We also conducted another little research project which isn't earthshaking, but I think rather intriguing. I asked a friend of mine who is 6'0" tall and of medium, slender build to dress in a dark suit and tie. We took him downtown to a sidewalk construction site on a busy day. The site was such as to force people into a single file wooden walkway. We then asked him to time his arrival at the same time of another male and to stop and offer the other man priority on the walkway.

We positioned ourselves so as to numerically record whether the man took priority or offered my friend priority in return. If he did so, my buddy was to take that priority and not offer again. This part was scientific but I also recorded something which I admit was quite subjective—but I attempted to be fair. I tried to judge the other person's facial expression as sorrowful, disgusted, bland, happy or very respectful. (This is obviously not science.)

In any event, my comrade did this "stunt" to 100 men. A whopping 82 returned his offer of priority ("No, you go ahead") either verbally or by headnod. And sixty of those 82 did so with what I interpreted as respect in their eyes and face.

He then did our same "trick" on 100 women of all sizes and ages. Even though women have culturally learned to go first, 42 still gave him first priority—and 90 seemed to me to have happy or respectful faces turned toward him whichever decision they made.

The very next day I asked a friend of mine who is approximately 60 lbs. overweight to do the EXACT same thing. He also is 6'0" tall and also wore a dark suit and tie. Of 100 men, only 58 returned his offer to go ahead, as opposed to 82 with my slender friend. Of those 58, at least 20 seemed to possess an obviously disgusted look as though he had inconvenienced them and 22, it appeared to me, had an expression of "you go first because I feel sorry for you." Their eyes dropped and their facial expressions were subdued. Of the women, only 12 didn't immediately take the offered priority. Of those 12 who returned priority, all 12 possessed what I saw as an expression of "feeling sorry for you." That I cannot prove, but I do know in my own mind it was not a look of instinctive respect or admiration. I do know that much psychology. In any event, it was easy to discern that the slender man was afforded much more respect by most strangers than was the obese man. If you feel that our research was faulty or bias, I urge you to conduct similar research.

SALES

We selected four pictures of persons overweight by approximately 30 lbs. One was a young woman in her mid-twenties; one of a man the same age; one of a middle-aged man; one of a middle-aged woman. We then produced four pictures of slim and trim men and women the same age.

We pledge to you (on my father's grave?) that in the name of science, we carefully attempted to make certain that they were equally dressed; equally groomed; of similar looks; and with the same facial expressions (pleasant smiles).

We took those pictures to 100 purchasing officers of companies picked at random and asked their "gut reaction" (five seconds to make the choice) as to which of the people they would most apt, all else being equal, buy a product from.

And we did something very interesting at this point. We mixed and matched obese with slender. For example, we showed each person 16 combinations—young obese male vs. young slender male; young obese male vs. older slender female, etc.

Upon completion, we had 1600 responses of various types of male and female obese salesmen vs. a variety of bi-gender slender salesmen. 73% of the purchasing agents selected the slender! That is highly significant three out of four statistic!

Now if my research is even close to reliable (you are obviously free to conduct your own), then either overweight sales people should consider losing weight—especially if you're a young person going into sales and haven't established your territory yet—or obesity groups had better petition the Supreme Court to include "or body type" to the law which states we can't discriminate because of race, religion, sex, etc. As a group, at least, it would certainly appear that obese people are just not going to be as effective in the "market place" as are slender persons.

SCHOOL ADMINISTRATORS

We took our picture test to 100 randomly selected school administrators and asked them to select which persons they would hire for a variety of teaching positions—again assuming that ALL other factors were equal, including degrees, experience, references and interviewing abilities. Eighty-three of the 100 selected slim, trim people. Of the 17 who selected hefty candidates, 12 were themselves overtly overweight. Though a few overweight administrators selected slender teachers, absolutely NO slender administrators picked fat persons. Again, if you are an obese teaching candidate, you might be wise to consider a school system with a "heavyweight" administrator at the top.

PARENTS OF STUDENTS

We took our photo album to 200 parents and asked them, "Which teacher(s) would you most want to teach your child in school—ALL else being equal?" We selected randomly 100 parents of elementary children and 100 of secondary school students. Of the elementary, 77 of 100 pointed to non-obese pictures. Of the secondary, 86 of 100 desired the slender candidates. Are you beginning to "get the PICTURE," too?

CONCLUDING STATEMENT ON RESEARCH

The evidence seems quite clear, at least to me, that America just doesn't find obesity to its liking very much. And this is quite ironic since we have such a high percentage of obese people.

It also seems evident that the generalized respect factor for highly overweight people is not as high as for the slender segment of our population. They seem to suffer from the "Rodney Dangerfield Syndrome." It may be unfortunate that this is so—and obese people may not like what they are reading here—but it appears to nevertheless be a "truism."

It is my opinion that there is a deep moral factor here growing from our Judaic-Christian roots. That is, we find objectionable the excess indulgence and lack of discipline that gross obesity almost always represents. I have a feeling that we could utilize truth serum, polygraph devices and pupillametrics and discover that even MOST obese people abhor obesity in others—as well as themselves. But this I know for dead certain, I spent 20 prime years of my life grossly overweight and I'll always regret that—though I spend little time wallowing in the past. AND I WILL PAY ANY PRICE TO MAKE CERTAIN THAT NEITHER I NOR MY CHILDREN ARE EVER FAT AGAIN!

It is not my intention here to condone said discrimination and preferential treatment. Perhaps obsessive-compulsive eaters should initiate the N.A.A.O.P.—The National Association for the Advancement of Obese People. Nevertheless, it appears to be an instinctive or cultural fact that grossly overweight people—in most areas of life—have the deck stacked against them. So it is for you to decide if you want to play the game (and life has always been just that—a game of hide and seek; a game of cops and robbers; a game of deception; a game of drama and theatre; a game of Russian roulette; and a game of monopoly) against a stacked deck. I never liked to do it in poker and I finally decided I didn't enjoy doing it in the game of obesity vs. success. In a significant number of instances, fat is an obstacle to success and happiness. I have probably "over-killed" that point in the first part of this book but it must sink in to you—as it had to for me—before we can proceed with a viable program.

HAVE YOU GIVEN UP?

It is quite obvious that many obsessive-compulsive foodaholics have given up and given in to their condition. They are no longer success oriented people—neither in their desire to be successful in losing weight or their desire to be successful in any other area of life. Just like their alcoholic "cousin," their entire life is built around their next meal. If they get 10 miles away from a restaurant, they undergo a panic attack. If you have given up, as did some members of my own family, then the remainder of this book is not for you. Because this book is an over-all growth and development book—and there is only one way you want to grow.

PART II

THE
JERRY L.
WALKE
PROGRAM

CHAPTER SIX

First, Let Me Be Honest

I just mentioned a 90% success rate of the persons with whom I work on a one-to-one basis. This is very high incidence of success. But I am not foolish enough to believe that 90% of you reading this book will be successful in conquering foodaholism, losing weight, and keeping it off. In fact, the rate will not be nearly so high. Why?

Well, I've been an educator and a counselor for many years. And I know that simply "reading a book" will not be sufficient for some of you to understand the magnitude of your problem and to internalize the principles involved in attacking (and changing/curing) the problem. Many of you simply will not understand or comprehend the process even though I've very much simplified it in this book; others of you will simply "pass off" the concepts; some of you don't really, down-deep (unconsciously) want to lose weight—you only pay lip-service to it and try to convince yourself and others; quite a few of you will even label my various steps (carefully devised over many years) as "silly and dumb;" and finally, many of you will not follow my recommended program because your spouse or fiance does not really want you to lose weight.

Let me take a moment to explain a strange phenomenon I've witnessed over many years of working with obese people. As a teacher of psychology for two decades, I understand the underlying motivations of this phenomenon, but as a human being I find it mystifying and incomprehensible. That is, it is a fact that many husbands will continually fight against their wives' efforts to lose weight and many wives continually strive to keep their husbands fattened hogs at the trough.

One would think that a husband would rejoice in his wife's weight loss program and renewed self-concept, energy, and achievement motivation. But far too often, such is not the case. The husband will deviously block almost every avenue she travels toward slenderness and will incessantly tempt her back into obsessive-compulsive eating patterns. HE ACTUALLY WANTS HER TO BE FAT!

We could get into some very deep psychology as to why this phenomenon persists, but suffice it to say that mostly it stems from the fact that he has the basic insecurity that A) her rebuilt self-image will cause her to grow and develop **BEYOND** him; and B) her slenderness and the accompanying attractiveness will present new competition to him and that she might "find someone else." Therefore his rationalized battle cry almost always becomes "Well, I like heavy women and I like you to be my little chicken dumpling."

As a counselor, I know the value of the "human element." That is, the presence of an empathetic person—in a one-to-one relationship—who will work with you on these principles and who TRULY CARES that you lose weight and keep it off. This empathetic relationship is a major part of counseling—as well as most forms of psychotherapy. It is highly significant and must not be discounted. This book in front of you does not, and CANNOT, substitute for the presence of a trained and caring person (such as me), even though I have tried my best to write this book in a very personal manner to you.

Now, having admitted the above, let me make two very important statements:

1) Those of you who read this book with deep conscientiousness and comprehension (that is, to "internalize" it) will still be successful in effecting this important change in your life. But you must truly want to win (see below). Read this book at least twice!

2) Possibly the best advice (I detest that word, don't you? How about the best recommendation) I'll give to you: Have someone else that you know truly cares for you—a wife, husband, friend, relative, lover, etc.—also read this book and ask them if they will "ride herd" on you for a few months until you have mastered/internalized the techniques. That is the amount of time I empathetically "journey" with my clients and it is sufficient time. If you're not truly serious about losing weight, then Jesus Christ himself can never help you. My father, and many other good Christian foodaholics, have proved that beyond a shadow of a doubt. I'll discuss this in more detail later, also.

Make no mistake, you can only make all these changes yourself, as is true of all things in your life. "If it's going to be done, you must do it." But it is a universal truth that the presence of an allied other, an other who likes you and cares for you, is an invaluable asset in this process. To be completely honest, with all my knowledge and expertise, I still was greatly aided by a "helpmate"—in my case, a registered nurse, trained vegetarian named Angela Yvonne Whitt, who worked beside me for six months, loved me very much, and deeply cared that I lost weight and took pride in my appearance.

She saved my life—certainly emotionally, and probably literally physically. Because I was truly a severe foodaholic and was heading for a quick gravesite!

I NEVER MET AN ATHLETE WHO DIDN'T WANT TO WIN!

Permit me here to present a small—but very important—PARABLE to you. This parable, like any good parable, applies to any achivement situation in life, whether it be weight loss, becoming wealthy, overcoming shyness, winning athletic contests or whatever.

You may, or may not, realize that I, along with my teaching, psychology work, and speaking/lecturing, was also a college coach for many years—most of them as a basketball coach. During that time, I never met or coached an athlete who didn't say that he LOVED to win. They constantly made such statements as "Man, I want to win badly" and "I hate to lose—just can't stand it." And when they won, they were jubilant. And when they lost, they were dejected. They cried, bitched, moaned, groaned, sat with towels over their heads, etc. So, on the surface (consciously), it appeared that they were telling the truth: They loved winning and hated losing. They truly believed it themselves and they expected you to, also. It all sounded good and made them feel good about themselves, I'm sure.

But do you know, in all those years, I personally only coached one—yes, ONE—athlete who really, truly proved that he meant it. Most of the rest either just paid lip service to winning or meant it only about 75%—and 75% is not too bad. That was enough to make my teams successful. But only ONE, a young man named Nick Mescher really actually loved to win—and constantly proved it. Since you do not know Nick Mescher, you need only picture in your mind Pete Rose or John Havlicek. They are the classic "winners" of my era and yours.

Let's take a look at the others, whose words sounded so impressive. They would continually exhibit at least one—sometimes all—of the following characteristics: They would often come to practice late and sometimes miss altogether; they would loaf in our various drills, saving themselves for scrimmages; they wouldn't push themselves in practice or conditioning drills; they would train poorly or stay up very late the night before games if not closely policed; they wouldn't dive on the floor for loose balls—even at crucial times in the game; they wouldn't "draw the charge" on a man driving to the basket; they wouldn't block their man off the backboards while rebounding, etc., etc., ad infinitum.

In short, they wouldn't do all the LITTLE THINGS that we teach/coach that permitted them to win (remember this message carefully). Yet, when we lost, they verbalized "I hate to lose" and went thru their "tough loss" ritual. I repeat, it sounded good, but as a coach I knew better, didn't I? Only impressive lip service. Nick Mescher, like the rare Pete Rose's and John Havlicek's, literally did EVERYTHING it took to win at all times. True winners!

Now the message here is quite clear. Only you can answer the following questions, and only your ACTIONS can tell you whether or not you're telling the truth—or simply fooling yourself and lying to yourself: Are you REALLY wanting to cure your foodaholism? Are you REALLY wanting to lose weight and keep it off? Are you ready to get your butt in gear (take actions to back your mouth)? As the Appalachian hillbillies like to say "Are you going to fish or cut bait?" Directly to the point, "Are you going to defecate? If not, get off the pot!"

NOW YOU MUST BE HONEST!

I have each of my clients sign a contract before I will work with him/her. This contract has absolutely nothing to do with money and, obviously, is not a legal, binding contract. But I do impress upon them that it is a morally, ethically binding contract and tell them not to sign it unless they TRULY mean it—so as to not waste their time and money, and my time.

Though you need not sign a contract with me, you are wasting your time reading further in this book unless you agree to the following: I AM ADMITTEDLY A FOODAHOLIC—A CONFIRMED OBSESSIVE-COMPULSIVE EATER. I NO LONGER WISH TO BE A FOODAHOLIC, AS OF THIS MOMENT, AND I WILL FOLLOW ALL OF DR. JERRY L. WALKE'S PRINCIPLES AND RECOMMENDATIONS. I TRULY DESIRE TO BE SLENDER THE REMAINDER OF MY LIFE AND TO CHANGE MY ENTIRE LIFESTYLE FOR THE BETTER. MY LIFE OF OBESITY IS OVER, PLACED IN MY PAST FOREVER!!! This commitment must be made to yourself—and me—before you go any further. You cannot change any behavior on your own, and very little can be changed for you, until you have recognized said behavior in yourself (Socrates' "Know thyself") and have a deep desire to change it. (The major basis of Carl Rogers' client-centered therapy).

The above is the basic concept of Alcoholics Anonymous and is just as relevant to foodaholism. Your problem is severe. It is, in a manner of speaking, a form of mental/emotional pathology (doesn't mean you're "crazy") and you must freely and unashamedly admit all this in order to structure a plan of action for "cure." You have, in all probability, rationalized your dietary behavior for years, as do most grossly overweight people. Even worse, you probably have internalized your emotional need to eat so deeply that it is simply a part of your lifestyle.

THE SCORPION PARABLE

I remember a story my grandfather told me when I was a young boy. Actually, the story is about people who have an internalized, Freudian pattern of aggression and destructiveness, but it is applicable here because it depicts the nature of unconscious motivation toward obsessive-compulsive eating just mentioned.

A turtle was preparing to swim across a creek (pronounced "crick" here in Appalachia). Suddenly, a scorpion appeared on the scene and asked pleadingly, "Mr. Turtle, may I ride across the stream on your back? We scorpions can't swim, you know."

"No way," said the turtle. "You'll zonk me with that big stinger of yours when I get out in the middle of the stream and I'll drown."

"Oh, come now!" responded the scorpion with sincerity dripping from his voice, "Use your head, turtle man, I wouldn't sting you in the middle of the stream, I can't swim, remember? Therefore, if you drown, I also would drown. I'm not that stupid."

"Oh, yeh," the turtle answered meekly, "I hadn't thought of that. C'mon, jump on and I'll take you to the other side."

Well, you guessed it, the turtle and his poison passenger got out in the middle of the stream and "ZONK!"—the scorpion plunged his stinger "clean through" the turtle's shell. The poison soon began to paralyze the tortoise's nervous system and he began to sink. As he was slowly going under, he looked up at his brutal assailant and asked, "Why did you do it, Mr. Scorpion? You can't swim and now you, too, shall die."

I know it turtle, ol' buddy, "He stated with a perplexed look on his face and in his eyes. But I just couldn't help myself. You see, it's just my nature!"

And, in all probability, the same is true of your self-destructive eating patterns. But, make no mistake. NATURE CAN BE CHANGED!

You're in the gutter, and you will never get out until you come to the full realization that you are there. You are destined, otherwise, to wallow in your own fat forever—or at least fluctuate like an elevator weight-wise. If you believe otherwise, you're only dreaming. Celebrity diets; U. S. Military diets; grapefruit juice diets; high protein diets; National Enquirer diets; vegetarian diets; exercise; jazzercise; swimmercize programs; etc., are, in themselves, a tragic waste of your time, effort and money.

Now, if you have made the above commitment, read on. If not, quit wasting your time with this book. Give it to someone else or use it to start a fire in your charcoal grill and "pig out" for the evening. However, if you have admitted the above, do NOT part with this book for a long time to come. It will be invaluable to you. You'll see why quite soon. Keep on reading!

THE LONG—BUT FUN AND CHALLENGING—JOURNEY

Now that you HAVE made the commitment, I have both bad news and good news for you. The bad news is that you have just begun a life-long journey. I have already informed you that crash diets and fad diets—and even organized Weight Watcher type programs—are largely ineffective. Only a complete change of habits, rituals, diet, and lifestyle will work. So, welcome to a new club, pilgrim! Meet and shake hands with a partner that will be with you from here into eternity.

The good news is two-fold:

1) After a given period of time—usually about six weeks, but it may range from immediately to three months in your case—the journey will become fun and challenging. Your entire life and lifestyle will change—for the better. What you see now as an insurmountable burden will become an intense joy in your life.

2) I (and hopefully your new-found, built-in "psychiatrist" that I recommended earlier) will accompany you on this journey for at least five months. I have carefully written the remainder of this book to attempt to relate to you as personally as possible even though, obviously, you probably don't know me at all. Therefore, as much as possible through written word, I'll be with you step-by-step, principle-by-principle. Your amateur "counselor" should also read this book at least twice and be prepared to also give you the psychological support you need and to "ride herd" on you until you are internalizing the steps necessary to success. If he/she loves you, he'll relish your "new-born" self and rejoice in your achievement.

You will make it. Almost all my people do! If you fail, your counselor fails—and I fail. If you succeed, your empathetic partner succeeds—and so do I. It is important to me that you DO succeed. I mean that! My file is filled with letters from hundreds of people who have and they are the chief source of my ego strength. The money is a distant second to me. Ask anyone who knows of the simple lifestyle I live—and enjoy. By the way, I have a very simple philosophy of money: You can always make it back working . . . and just wait until you read my thoughts on work.

One of the major thrusts of my life (career) on this earth is to reduce/eliminate foodaholism. I'll explain why later.

IMPORTANT PERSONAL NOTE!!

If you are to be "cured;" if my program is to work; you must follow EVERY step and assignment religiously. You must consider NOTHING to be trivial, silly or unnecessary. Do you understand? NOTHING! Every assignment (sound like a typical teacher, don't I?) must be fulfilled. If not, you will probably fail—and I will not take the responsbility. It has taken me many years to originate and develop this program and PLACE IT IN THE PROPER SEQUENCE. Therefore, everything counts! Disregard nothing! Ready to go?

CHAPTER SEVEN

Let Us Begin!

ASSIGNMENT #1

Every day, I said EVERY day, for the next three weeks, you must read the aforementioned "I am a foodaholic" admission entirely, and aloud. It must be internalized, even into the inner recesses of your cerebral cortex and limbic system (soon to be explained). The assignment is easy but must be fulfilled. Do it for (in order of importance) yourself, your counselor and me. Do not miss one day! Not one single day until your target weight is achieved. Do you understand?

NOTE!

If you do not fulfill every assignment faithfully, for whatever reason (excuse), then you are already telling yourself that you are simply like the athlete who SAYS he wants to win. Six weeks from now, if you have neglected any assignment, you have proven to yourself your true motives. Get rid of this book and head for the "Frig!" Your need to self-destruct simply overwhelmed this book.

BE COOL!

Whatever the cause(s) of your foodaholism—and you should have little or no concern of the causes as it serves little purpose—you did not develop your obsessive-compulsive food needs overnight and no program can solve them overnight. You can't solve the problem OVERNIGHT yourself by any words you utter or psychological commitment you make (with rare exceptions).

Most foodaholics search their entire lives for instantaneous and miraculous cures for their problem. This is why tabloid newspaper (Enquirer), diet books and fad diets (herbs, grapefruit, water diets, etc.) are multi-billion dollar businesses. Well, I'm sorry to inform you that that just ain't where it's at. Interestingly, the solution to your problem, as I'll show you, is relatively simple, but it does not and will not take place like a "salvation" at a Billy Graham Crusade. Instant salvation and Christianity at the altar is all well and good for religion, and I'll not take issue with it here. But it has not, and will not, work in the area of permanent weight loss and weight control. History has proved that beyond a shadow of a doubt. Leave the miracles to Billy and Oral. Which reminds me, if cancerous growths can be dried up *immediately* by faith healers and ulcers healed immediately, why is there no recorded case in history of fat being removed *immediately*. It is just as destructive and its instant removal should be an easy chore for Oral and his compadres. (Lest this be taken as a harsh criticism of faith healers, let me surprise you by affirming that actually faith healers do "heal" certain types of psychosomatic and hysteric maladies and, therefore, do represent a positive force in our society. By the way, psychiatrists and psychologists perform the same service. Only the modus operandi is different. That's why I've never completely understood the rift between the two fields). This is why I have noted that you will probably only begin to see results in six weeks to three months—and ONLY if you follow all principles and recommendations. So, for the next six weeks (at least), cool it! Don't expect miracles. They'll occur soon enough! Trust me!

LET'S TALK ABOUT THE SCALES!

To almost every dieter, the scales become an essential instrument. Most persons weigh themselves at least once daily and often more. Even a nationally known program such as Weight Watchers requires weekly (or more) trips to the scales. I contend, and will show, that this is a major error and even self-defeating. The scales are a major enemy to you in my program!

To weigh yourself regularly is exactly what you DON'T want to do. Why?

1) It serves to remind you that you are obese, a concept that I'll soon prove is the central "malpractice" of almost every weight loss program. We

(you and I) will be quickly working AWAY from that image, not toward it. So the scales become your mortal adversary.

2) Since one loses weight in spurts, and suffers many plateaus in which, no matter what one does, he won't lose weight, the constant use of scales becomes discouraging. Therefore, again, they become your foe and can cause you to "give up" in the early stages of my program. Avoid the scales as you would a Castro with bad breath.

So go ahead and weigh yourself now and record your weight. Also, set your "target" weight now—that minimum weight you desire to attain. Then, get rid of the scales. Forget them! At most, weigh yourself maybe once every six months. Since you are beginning a life-long journey, your weight at any given time means nothing, anyway. How many pounds you have lost in any given time span (day, week, month, year) is just as insignificant. Keep your buttocks off the scales!

THE "CHANGE" WE ARE SEEKING

The ultimate goal we foodaholics search for is quite simple, and one you have probably heard previously because it was first coined by Ben Franklin.

I just live to eat	*I simply eat to live*

this change must be made

We both know, of course, that even though it sounds so simple, attaining the above is difficult, right? Well, maybe so, maybe not! We'll see. The past eight years I have watched hundreds of people do it with the program presented in this book. Quite frankly, I think you'll be astounded at how easy the change above is to implement.

— IMPORTANT POINT —

If this alteration in your approach to food is not made, then all your efforts to lose weight and maintain that loss come only because of SELF-DISCIPLINE and WILL POWER. And, contrary to popular opinion, self-discipline and will power are seldom adequate in any long-term weight change. Shocking news to you possibly, but true! Some degree of self-discipline and will power will be important only in the beginning of my program. But the ultimate goal will be to erase the need of them altogether. Most diets and weight loss programs are simply exercises in frustration because they are based upon self-discipline and will power. As I'll show you, both simply keep reminding you that you're fat.

PEANUT BUTTER COOKIE PARABLE

Let me give you an example of where we are heading. I've already reached the "top of the mountain" and sit here proudly. Now you are going to scale it, also. One of the multitudinous tastes I was hooked on (literally, just like a drug addict) was hot, homemade peanut butter cookies. Anytime I was hungry and saw them, even if only in a picture, "GET YOUR CHILDREN OFF THE STREET, here comes Jerry!" And once I tasted the first one, "Katy, bar the door." I either ate them all or ate until I was sick (both physically and emotionally—because of the guilt and shame I felt because I had just pigged out). Does all this sound familiar with at least one taste (probably many more) you crave/desire (at this point, select YOUR very favorite taste)?

Most diet programs are unsuccessful simply because they move you to a point where you still desire the peanut butter cookies (substitute your favorite taste) but resist them—maybe—because of self-discipline and will power. Only rarely do you meet a confirmed foodaholic who can sustain that practice over a long period of time. Believe me, it's not the way to go. I can NOW have a plate of peanut butter cookies set down before me and have absolutely no desire for them. It would be one thing to say what I just did to YOU or try to convince YOU, but I can honestly say to myself that I have no down-deep, internalized desire for even one of those cookies. Periodically, maybe once every six months, I'll eat one—yes, just ONE—to prove to myself that I'm not being neurotic (obsessive-compulsive) about NOT eating. A neurosis is a neurosis, whether used positively or negatively. I've probably eaten sweets maybe six times in the past four years. And then only to taste them minimally, usually one piece. I truly have no desire for refined sugar of any type. The sugar industry would go broke quickly if they had to depend on Jerry L. Walke. They consider me a mortal enemy—just as I do them! They've killed far more people than cocaine and heroin dealers, drunken drivers, breweries and distilleries, tobacco companies and Union Carbide all combined. I wonder why the U. S. Government and public hasn't caught onto them yet and forced them to put warning labels on ALL their products: "Excessive use of this product can be extremely hazardous to your health. It has been proven to cause death in laboratory rats—oops, humans."

Whoops, back on my soapbox, again! Back to reality. You MUST make the psychological change from living to eat to eating to live and you MUST reach the "mountaintop" of moving past self-discipline and will power to the point of simply—and honestly—having no desire for the peanut butter cookies. We are getting nearer to the point of where I'll show you how to do it.

ASSIGNMENT #2

QUIT TALKING ABOUT FOOD

As soon as you have completed reading this book (preferably twice), your second assignment is to no longer discuss food or at least as seldom as possible. Naturally, you have to make such statements as "It's time to eat," etc. But other than these survival statements, cease and desist from discussing food, diets, calories, obesity, menus, etc. The reason for this is exactly the same as forgetting about the scales. Discussing all the above things reminds you that you are fat and/or that you are presently hungry. This process is going to be a life-long one anyway, so there is no need to talk about (or even think about) the whole thing. As you'll see soon, you're only negatively programming yourself, literally dooming yourself to failure.

I laugh (or cry) when I see someone (often times a psychologist) recommend or practice, the principle of placing a picture of their obese self on the refrigerator door or even have the refrigerator door tripping a tape recording when opened saying something like "Are you eating again, Fatso?" Methods such as these are not only useless, they serve to promote and reinforce your foodaholic-ism and condition you eventually to regain any loss you might make (through self-discipline, I remind you).

So, as soon as you finish this book, let's forget food-talk, O.K.? Remember, all my principles, no matter how trivial sounding to you, are essential. Do your assignments! (Sound like a typical teacher again, huh?).

There is flat-out no need to discuss calories, weight, diets, fattening foods, non-fattening foods, etc. It's kind of like the person who must keep reminding you over and over how Christian they are and it soon becomes obvious that they're trying harder to convince themseles than they are you.

HOW ABOUT "BREAK-OVERS?"

At least for the next six weeks to three months, you are in all probability, going to break-over and "pig out" in your eating ritual. You might not, if you have enough will power—or better labeled "won't power"—and you will admittedly be operating on will power during this time. But, if you are a typical foodaholic, your obsession will get the best of you for a while.

No sweat! Don't worry about it for now. Just try your best, for the time being, not to push the "panic button" when you break-over and completely bloat yourself, and you know exactly what I mean by "bloat." You've had that experience/feeling many times. Don't permit a break-over to become a binge! Try to grab hold of your wrist tightly (literally) and say to yourself, "O.K., I've broken over now, but don't go wild and bloat yourself, Dummy."

Later on, as the entire program begins to take effect, you won't have to worry about it, anyway. But, in the meantime, try to use your self-discipline not to break-over, and if you DO then try not to go "hog wild"—an appropriate slang term. That's assignment #3.

STATING THE OBVIOUS

The following is a painfully obvious, elementary statement, but it must be made at this point nevertheless:

A) In order to lose weight, on any given day you must take in fewer calories than you burn up, and;

B) In order to maintain any weight loss, you must take in the same number of calories you burn up, and;

C) Any given day you take in more calories than you burn up, you will gain weight.

Barring some major illness, the above will be true the remainder of your life.

I realize that you already know all this. So why state it here? Well, it's a reminder that, if you are grossly overweight (remember, 30 lbs. or more), then you probably have a cellular body make-up and corresponding metabolic rate that easily converts food substances into body tissue (fat). In other words, if you eat 2,001 calories on a given day and only burn up 2,000, that one calorie will become fat—and you are destined to live with that burden the rest of your days on this earth. This is exactly why it will do you no good to think in terms of "I'll diet for a while and then go back to eating whatever I wish." As stated previously, that constant "elevator trip" is simply a long, lonely road to nowhere—and 97% of American dieters think EXACTLY that way.

Therefore, even though A,B,C, above are quite obvious, you might as well commit them to memory and lock them forever in your brain/computer right now. God, heredity, universal law or whatever dealt you a "bad hand" in terms of body style. How heavenly it would be to be a foodaholic with an eternally slender (ectomorph) body. But you ain't got one, Mr./Ms. endomorph-mesomorph! But we'll learn together, you and I, to thumb our nose at heredity and universal laws of probability. To heck with 'em! Who needs an ectomorph body anyway? We'll create one.

SO, WHAT ABOUT YOUR DIET!

What is a good diet program for you? Do you wish to become a vegetarian? Do you go on a Weight Watcher-type program? High protein? Stillman's Water diet? Jane Fonda's program? One your doctor recommends? One from National Enquirer? Or Ladies Home Journal?

I don't really give a damn, Scarlet. And you don't need to be concerned about it right now either. Just give us a little time together and the type of diet you decide upon will just naturally take care of itself. Because I can't practice medicine, I must make a standard comment that you should consult your physician before you undertake any diet and/or exercise program. But, other than that, do not even concern yourself with it for a while. You will soon seek and select a program in a "mysterious" manner. You'll see. And, ah how you are going to enjoy your "mysterious" thinking.

During the interim, just begin to use whatever will power you possess to simply reduce portions of whatever diet you're on now. If you usually eat two pieces of cake for dessert or one giant piece, try to eat only a small sliver. You know what I mean. You've probably been doing it off and on all your life, and watching the fat go "off and on" all the while. Assignment #4—Begin to cut portions and give it your best shot (remember, without getting "all shook up" about break-overs).

ASSIGNMENT #5

EAT SLOW!

95% of obsessive-compulsive eaters eat embarrassingly fast. They usually wolf it down so quickly that they are a social embarrassment to themselves and those around them. In addition, they defeat their major purpose as a foodaholic—that is, they don't even end up enjoying what they sat down to enjoy. A meal becomes a job (work) and a race. It even becomes a war because they attack the food with a vengeance. And, as in any war, to the victor belongs the spoils—in this case, the guilt that follows your ravaging carnage.

I was in a restaurant just a few days ago and observed a scene that I've seen often—and participated in just as often. Three women (just as easily could have been men) who were grossly overweight went through a six-course meal—cocktails, appetizers, salad, soup, main dish and dessert—in ten minutes! And it would have been faster if the waitress could have hauled it to them quicker. I am truly not exaggerating. It was nerve wracking to witness.

I was sitting in the bar area with two friends, both non-foodaholics and they could not believe what they were seeing. We were elevated above the dining area and, therefore, had a bird's eye view of the "carnage." And speaking as a professor of psychology, it was carnage in the truest sense—that is, not only was it carnivorous, but also a carnal sex ritual in which these three women were releasing their libido (getting their "rocks off") in their "pillage" of that food. Make no mistake, a great deal of obsessive-compulsive eating is an aggressive sex ritual.

My two friends were shocked—and quite humored. And I said to them, "You could never comprehend what those three women are doing, feeling, and enduring. But I can! Please do not laugh at them or condemn them. They are highly similar to the skid row bum in the gutter. Pity them and be filled with compassion."

At this point, I have a need to also tell you about a woman with whom I have taught. She is a very nice woman and highly intelligent. I like her very much though she has always been somewhat aloof and distant to me. It might be because she is extremely, extremely obese and she knows I've become a specialist (authority?) in weight loss—weight control. Let's call her Prudi (not her name). I think the reason I'm so attracted to her (just human to human) is that she reminds me of my favorite cousin Diane. Diane was equally suffering from gross obesity; they even look alike; Diane was also an exellent teacher; and she was also highly intelligent and creative. The world was hers for the taking—just as it is for Prudi. But you notice that I keep using the word "was." My cousin, Diane, died at age 31 purely from over eating. She literally ate herself to death. What a tragic waste of human-ness.

Prudi is traveling the same road and I would so much like to help in altering her course. I hope she reads this book and "digests" its contents. That alone would make all my time, effort, blood, sweat and tears poured into this book worthwhile. But to the point: two weeks ago I watched (without her knowledge) Prudi inhale a gigantic pizza and three large colas in less than five minutes. So help me, I am not exaggerating. Less than five minutes. There could absolutely not be any emotional satisfaction in such a carnage. In fact, to the contrary, only destruction and emotional scar tissue were achieved.

Back to assignment #5. Begin to slow down in your eating. Make a rule of laying down your utensil or sandwich or piece of celery, etc. between EVERY bite. Even eat exaggeratedly slow for a while. Chew slow, swallow slow, whatever. Just don't wolf it down. Good lovers go slow. And good eaters should go slow also. Follow the advice of that old country song "Give Me A Lover (Eater) With A Slow Hand."

EMOTIONAL FOOD SATISFACTION IS ALL RELATIVE

You must next fully understand that obsessive-compulsive eating is fulfilling very deep emotional needs—while, of course, causing additional serious emotional problems. It's a very vicious, self-perpetuating cycle, much like a snowball going down a mountain. Yes, foodaholism is very much of an emotional nature. This is precisely why we continually eat even FAR after we have satisfied all hunger needs within the survival/hunger system of the R-complex (Hindbrain). Then the emotions in the Limbic System of the midbrain take over. However, emotional food satisfaction is very relative, and you can train/teach/condition yourself to gain equal satisfaction from a low-calorie food as much as a high calorie food. The suggestion (assignment) I'll make to you now is NOT a major part of my program, but it is nevertheless, a solid, proven practice that has helped me, and many others, immensely.

Remember assignment –5—EAT SLOW! Now, combined with that, try this, assignment #6. Let's go back to my peanut butter cookies for a moment. Let us say that I also enjoy raw broccoli dipped in a low calorie ranch dressing—which I do. I go to the kitchen or restaurant and fix (order) a serving of same. At this point, I initiate a ritual which will give me equal emotional satisfaction to the cookies. You won't think so at this time, I'm sure, but soon it will work for you. Right now, you will say to me "that there is no way, absolutely no way, that I can get the same satisfaction from a salad I enjoy as I can from a steak and fries." Oh, yes you can, EMOTIONALLY. It's all relative! I guarantee you it will happen if you follow my program conscientiously.

. . . . . MY RITUAL:

A) I first spread the serving out, even break it into smaller portions, so that I can fulfill the emotional need of "Oh, man, look how much I have to eat. Wow!" Of course, I'm playing a game with myself—fooling myself—but then obsessive-compulsive eating is ALL a mental game of deception anyway, isn't it?

B) Eat slow! Make the emotional satisfaction last, and last, and last!

C. With each bite, since you like this particular food anyhow, say to yourself (even aloud if you're alone): "Oh, is this good;" "Man, this is great;" "This is the best food I've ever eaten;" etc. and say all this with emotional/deep feeling. Get the point? Of course, I know the tastes are different, but you'll soon learn to pacify the Limbic System (the midbrain, where the emotions are housed) equally with broccoli as much as with peanut butter cookies. Sounds stupid? I told you earlier that no part of this program is, even this minor part. I can assure you that I now get MORE satisfaction from broccoli/dip than I do peanut butter cookies. So can you, with a little practice of the above ritual. It will not happen overnight, but then, your present pattern of eating didn't develop instantaneously either, remember?

MY DIET

I will now give you the diet that has worked for me—free of charge. You and/or your physician, can decide if it is the proper diet for you. You must select what is comfortable for you and your life style, and what you select is of little concern to me. Mine has worked for me; permitted me to lose 100 lbs. in the past four years; and feel better at 46 years old than I did at 23. So I'm sold on it. "Borrow" it if you like:

A) In the morning I drink a large glass of water and large glass of pure fruit juice or V-8 (my favorite) juice. If fruit, orange juice is certainly my choice. I drink these liquids while taking megavitamins and minerals and I'm flat-out sold on megavitamins dosages. Following is my intake:

1) Multi-vitamin pill (One-A-Day, plus iron)

2) Iron pill (Nature Made)

3) Gelatin capsules (Revco)

4) Vitamin A and D pill (Super X)

5) Vitamin B complex (Schiff)

6) KLBG pill (Nature's Bounty)

7) Three Vitamin E pills (100 I.U.) (Nature's Bounty)

8) Two Vitamin C pills (100 I.U.) (Nature's Bounty)

9) One protein pill (Nature's Blend)

10) One potassium pill (Plus)

11) One zinc pill (Nature's Blend)

B) I then work all day with only a light salad or raw vegetables for lunch.

C) After work, usually around 4:00 p.m., I eat raw fruits and vegetables and low cholesterol cheeses. Sometimes I'll dip my vegetables in a low calorie dip, sometimes not.

D) At the same time, I oftentimes drink beer, but only sparingly. I have gone thru two or three difficult periods in my life when I drank heavier, but now I only partake of alcohol VERY SPARINGLY—and we can scientifically prove that doing so is actually quite healthy. You'll have to follow your own instincts and morality on beer/alcohol. I, personally, never had a single drink until I was 30 years old, mainly because I was raised in a teetotaler Methodist home. Quite frankly, in my case, I think my non-partaking was an error. I was too rigid with myself and this rigidity caused me to endure much discomfort. Obviously, heavy drinking is dangerous both to others and self and I do NOT condone it. I now am a firm believer in moderation and limit my alcohol intake quite carefully.

To explain quickly, I have always been a high-anxiety, high body tension person. I do not take any drugs—and never did—except alcohol. Beer has a tranquilizing effect on me that relaxes my tension and, therefore, permits me to enjoy daily life more. I will never make any apologies for the above. Because I am a highly visible person who is in the public eye often, I've had to endure a reputation that I drink heavier than I do. It is not so!

E) At approximately 8:00 - 9:00 p.m., I either eat a vegetarian meal; or seafood meal; or on rare occasions a steak/roast beef if prepared without grease or cholesterol. I avoid fat meat and seldom eat bread or butter of any type. Though I am not basically a beef/pork person, and seldom eat them, I do feel that some fast food restaurants (such as Bonanza) are beginning to prepare their beef in a much healthier manner. Hopefully, books such as mine will continue to pressure restaurants and fast food franchises to be more responsible in their menus and preparation of food.

I retire usually around midnight—arise usually at 6:30.

SO WHAT
ABOUT YOUR EXERCISE PROGRAM?

There is no question that a regular exercise regimen is going to have to be part of your lifestyle. You might as well settle that in your mind right now and come to terms with it. This may seem like a life sentence to prison if you are anti-exercise like most grossly overweight, foodaholic persons, but you will find that, once my entire program "package" begins to take effect, vigorous exercise actually will become FUN for you. Given the body styles you and I are "stuck" with, we cannot lose weight (short of starvation), keep it off, and regain body definition (I'll discuss this soon) without a regular—not necessarily daily, but preferably—exercise program.

Just as with diet discussions earlier, I must first state that no exercise program should be undertaken without a complete physical exam and consultation with your physician. So much for my legal duties. And, just as before with diet, it makes little difference, at this time, what your exercise program is. Don't even worry about it at this time. "Mysterious thinking" (soon to be defined) will quickly lead you to a good program.

For the present (if your doctor approves), just begin walking every day until you are tired—not exhausted. This walking should be done in addition to your work, no matter how much walking you do on the job, and it should be recreational walking, that is, to observe with all your senses and to "stop and smell the roses." When you finish walking, exercise vigorously in any manner you wish until you are breathing hard and perspiring profusely, even if it only takes a few minutes to do so. That's enough for now. You'll soon develop, evolve, and gravitate toward a program most suited for your lifestyle and enjoyment. You will "mysteriously" seek a program of exercise that is recreation for you and not work. That program will then be a part of your lifestyle.

MY EXERCISE PROGRAM

I presented you my diet earlier and said that you could "borrow" it if you desired. The same is true with my exercise program, but it is not as likely you would wish to have it since there are so many diverse ways to exercise and you should select some that are fun and challenging to you so that you don't consider them "laborious work." I am also a great believer in a variety of activities so that you "work-out" in some manner almost every day, only periodically taking a day off so as not to become "neurotic" about the whole thing. The sky is the limit here; tennis, golf, jogging, walking, jazzercise, calisthenics, karate, etc. The list is almost endless.

I have a variety of activities in which I participate, but let me give you a typical week in my exercise life, keeping in mind that I am a teacher and writer—both very sedentary activities: In the beginning, in my case over a year, I jogged EVERY day. You must realize that my obsession with EVERY DAY was actually just another manifestation of obsessive-compulsive behavior which led to my negative eating habits, but at least jogging was a more positive "channeling" of same. This every day jogging was done purely through self-discipline and, as already stated, self-discipline and will power are simply not sufficient in the long run. Actually, I detested jogging, and still do, but I'll show you later how jogging "mysteriously" evolved in my program.

Presently, I jog about three times weekly, ranging from a minimum of two miles to a maximum of 14 miles. When I first began, I could not go one block, and was ashamed of how far I had permitted my body and its systems to deteriorate. I still hate each step of the way, quite frankly, but love the high feeling I know I'll experience when finished. Many joggers testify to the fact that they receive a "high" WHILE jogging. I've experienced it on rare occasions—but darn rare.

I work out on Nautilus equipment four times weekly. This I enjoy although I began on free weights and found those non-enjoyable but rewarding in the body definition they gave me. I'll discuss "body definition" next. In any event, Nautilus gives me the same body definition and I recommend it very highly.

I play racquetball at least four times weekly (usually BEFORE Nautilus) and I flat-out love the game. It is a great sport for both men and women because 1) you can get a good work-out quickly; 2) you have fun while getting that brisk work-out; 3) you can get in and out quickly—as opposed to tennis and golf; 4) it is not nearly as expensive as most sports; 5) maybe most important, you can learn to become at least a decent player in a relatively short span of time; and 6) it is a great release of aggressive and/or sexual energies which are so basic to obsessive-compulsive behavior—in our case, foodaholism.

I happen to be quite competitive and take a great delight in the fact that, even though I'm 46 years old, I can still beat most of the young "turks/studs"—one of the few sports in which an "old man" can still accomplish such. All this is such a Freudian sexual victory and it gives me identity and confidence—albeit minor and temporary. In short, it is a much better "getting rocks off" experience than inhaling a meal. Remember those three women I discussed previously.

Seasonally, I also periodically play golf and tennis, and I enjoy them both even though I'm not very good. I play both purely for fun and exercise and take neither too seriously, which I consider fortunate when I observe the behavior of most serious participants. They seem to make it work rather than fun.

I also do calisthenics once in a while (hate them) and jazzercises with TV (detest them also, but the womens' bodies do inspire me). For a 46 year old man, I'm now a fairly good "specimen" but I am not vain about it. I'll discuss the importance of non-vanity later.

So, assignment #7: begin exercise of some type and let it evolve and develop into YOUR program. I'll show you later how that will happen in a very natural manner.

BODY DEFINITION

If you are grossly overweight, you probably have little or no body definition. In other words, you probably stick out in all the wrong places and are "caved in" in all the wrong places. And you darn well don't need me to tell you where you most want to stick out and where you most want to be "caved in." Most of you are like I was a few years ago. You're "in shape" all right—pear-shaped!

I have noticed over the years that women, in particular, seem to lose weight from the neck down—men also to a lesser degree. This usually causes a problem for simple self-discipline dieters and might also in your case if we do not discuss it briefly.

As the entire program which follows starts to take hold and be effective, you will begin losing weight. However, there are some points where, if you're not aware of them, it is quite easy to become discouraged. One of these is the point described above—that we seem to lose weight from the neck down. Therefore, even after you have lost significant amounts of weight, you will probably still note that "My chest still sags;" "My lower stomach still sags;" "My hips and butt are still too big;" "My legs are still fat;" and/or "My calves and ankles are still too large."

These body areas are our most noticeable and we like to have them look as nice as possible (again, without reaching a point of vanity). You must realize this downward scheme of weight loss and further realize that it will take time and work to reach the desired appearance. But it WILL happen. Patience, jackass, patience! (Remember that old campire joke)? Your program is a lifetime program, anyway, and a lack of patience—the belief that everything must happen NOW—is indicative of the type of behavior pattern that led you to foodaholism in the first place. So, cool it, Mr./Ms. "neurotic mess!"

I've had quite a few women, in particular, who have lost significant amounts of weight and yet had lost almost none in their hips and thighs. This was most depressing to them until I informed them that this area would probably be the last to show positive results. They were very elated when soon after they found that the fat was beginning to melt away in those areas, also. So knowing the scheme and pattern of weight loss may help you not to become discouraged or frustrated.

FINAL NOTE

I have just presented you some excellent little tips and made some small, simple little assignments. Heed the tips and fulfill the assignments. We're on our way. However, we've only just begun. We're only warming up for the good stuff. Let us continue, together.

Admittedly, I was very tough on you the first three chapters. You will note that I've backed off a little the past four chapters. From this point onward, almost everything I teach (write) will be very positive in nature. I've found it necessary to "bop" people over the head and get their attention first. You might refer to it as "shock therapy," "reality therapy" or "directive counseling."

CHAPTER EIGHT

Self-Concept Psychology

THE KEYSTONE OF THE PROGRAM

Now we reach the major thrust of my program—that on which we'll "hang our hats"—in fact, all our smaller size clothes. Now we get down to nutcrackin' time! In the past 15 years, there has been a very strong emphasis on self-concept principles within the field of psychology. Hundreds of books have been written on the various aspects of and approaches to self-concept/self-image and its vast significance. During that time, the major thrust of my career has become self-concept psychology and I've attempted to take its basic structure and creatively formulate new theories and programs.

It's not that self-concept is new. The Bible refers to it often—especially in the New Testament—with such statements as "You must love others as yourself," etc., which implies what we now realize—that your ability to be intimate with others is directly relative to your love, acceptance, and intimacy with yourself. But it has only been in the past 15-20 years that we have fully understood just HOW IMPORTANT self-concept is and how much of a problem the lack of it is in this country (and world) today. Two important points:

1) Poor self-concept is by far the worst psychological problem in the world today. Sure, nuclear threat, crime, air and water pollution, cancer, starvation, war, etc., are all severe problems. But our true universal tragedy is that millions of humans just don't like themselves very well—and these people are destined to live lives of quiet desperation. And millions more just do not like themselves at all—and they are destined to live lives of quiet despondency. As a matter of fact, many of the above problems grow out of lack of wholesome self-image and the accompanying lack of ego stregnth (war is a prime example). People who do not like themselves much also do not like others much. Therefore, they consciously and/or unconsciously cause many, many problems for others.

2) The quality of life that you and I lead from today on to death will be directly relative to the degree of self-concept we possess. If you have solid and wholesome self-concept, your life will mostly be fun, challenging, and creative. If you don't like yourself very much, your life will, for the most part, be one of "quiet desperation" in which you simply go through the motions. If you don't like yourself at all, you are destined to live a life of quiet despondency and withdrawal. Therefore, self-concept is what it's all about, my fellow human. It is everything, and must be developed and nurtured carefully! As Sammy Davis, Jr. once sang: "I Can't Be Right For Somebody Else If I'm Not Right For Me."

THE FIVE BASIC
PRINCIPLES OF SELF-CONCEPT

There are five basic principles of self-concept psychology as I see it. Let's consider the first two together:

1) MOST people will perceive ("see") you as you perceive ("see") yourself, and

2) MOST people will treat you as you treat yourself.

There is no doubt in my mind that the two principles above are UNIVERSAL TRUTHS! You can apply any adjectives, verbs or adverbs you wish to the above two statements and they will prove to be so.

If you like (or love) yourself, MOST people will sense same and will also like (or love) you. If you don't like/love yourself, MOST people will take note instinctively and not like/love you either.

If you are aggressive with yourself (tough on yourself), MOST people will be aggressive with you.

If you are gentle with your self, MOST people will be gentle with you.

If you respect yourself, MOST people will respect you.

If you have pride in yourself and your appearance, MOST others will treat you and see you accordingly. We could go on, and on, and on. Apply any behavior pattern you desire. Now, the only word we must explain is the word "MOST." Wait a few minutes.

Assuming that principles #1 and #2 are even close to accurate—which they are—then the inverse must be true:

3) You will see MOST people as you view yourself, and

4) You will treat MOST people as you treat yourself.

If you are honest, you will see MOST people as trustworthy. If you are dishonest, you will see MOST people as dishonest. (Read the Watergate tape transcriptions).

If you truly see yourself as basically good and worthy, you will see (and treat) MOST others as good and worthy.

If you see yourself as a loving and intimate person, you will see MOST other people as loving and intimate. Conversely, if you see yourself as immature, unstable, "sick," dirty, sinful or whatever, you'll see most other people as immature, unstable, "sick," dirty, sinful or whatever. You can soon see that one must be careful he doesn't begin to deceive himself (play games with himself) because that person, therefore, who starts believing that most everyone is very sinful and evil might just be manifesting that he deeply and inwardly fears that he is sinful or evil—or would be given half a chance. Of course, we've known that for many years in the field of psychology. Sigmund Freud delineated that concept (reaction formation) very well. Actually, Shakespeare even did so long before Freud with his famous quote "Thou doth protesteth too much."

Again, we could list examples of these principles all night long in this book. But where many of us fall into the trap of wrong thinking is not understanding the meaning of the word "MOST." Let's take a closer look.

THE LASSIE PARABLE

We once owned a dog we named Lassie. There was nothing else to call her because she was a registered sable collie just as you saw for years in movies and on TV. She was beautiful and knew she was. That is, in the truest sense in human terms, she had an excellent, wholesome self-image.

All of you have also seen the cowering, whimpering, insecure, slinking, neurotic dog around your neighborhood at various times. The dog which, in human terms, obviously suffers (for whatever reason) from lack of self-concept. What happens to that dog? You know the answer. Most people mistreat the dog or at least run it away. They don't want it around. Most of the neighborhood kids yell "git" at it and/or hurl stones and insults at it. Of course, you (hopefully) and I treat it kindly and pet or feed it—but only because we feel sorry for it, no other reason. There is a message there somewhere.

Well, you know how collies instinctively seem to like children. So even though we had a fence around the yard, when the neighborhood kids were out playing, Lassie would often get excited and jump the fence.

Now what happened to those same kids who were mistreating the poor self-concept dog? You guessed it. They literally fought and begged to get Lassie to their group on their side of the street. They wanted her around and loved it when she was. A real message for us humans, too. At least, MOST of them wanted her around.

But I'm not stupid. My name might be Wimple, but it's not Simple. My name might be Willy, but it's not Silly. We must keep using the word "MOST" because I also knew that there were a couple of boys in the neighborhood who would still throw rocks or try to hurt Lassie anytime they had the opportunity. In other words, no matter how well she saw or treated herself, those two "scrotes" would try to mistreat her. But, you must understand, those two boys were the "problem" boys of the neighborhood—"emotionally disturbed" boys—and the term "emotionally disturbed" means just exactly what it says—that one or more of the human feelings is greatly exaggerated or non-exaggerated. Put more simply, one is labeled "emotionally disturbed" if one suffers from too much guilt or too little; too much depression or too little; or, in this case, too much AGGRESSION. The two boys in question here were highly aggressive, highly anti-social kids—commonly called juvenile delinquents—who enjoyed physically abusing ANY dog. The newest term in psychology is "assaultive." These young boys were assaultive youth who would, in all probability, become assaultive adults.

Of course, the same is true with humans. No matter how much a woman respects herself, there are still men waiting out there in hiding to throw her down, rip off her clothes, and rape her. But those are the "problem" people—the emotionally disturbed people—and they are a small minority. One must always be careful not to begin judging all of mankind based upon the small percentage of problem "scrotes." We must of course, be cautious and protect ourselves from them, but we must not fall into the trap of seeing all people thusly. When you do, YOU suffer the most.

If you see yourself as successful, MOST people will see you as successful, and work toward your success, but I already know there are those who will "rain on your parade" and work to tear down what you've built. But those are the "problem," emotionally disturbed persons and, I repeat, you must remember that they are a small minority.

The trap most of us fall into is that we begin judging the whole world based on that small minority and thus forget and lose the great advantage and worth of self-concept psychology. Let me give you a few typical examples:

A) So many times in my counseling career I've talked with women who have had a bad experience (or series of negative experiences) with some scoundrel of a man. They have been hurt and became bitter and now see all men as scoundrel "scrotes." Obviously, such is not true. But, amazingly, the moment they make this decision, the person who suffers most is them personally. Not only are they destined to a life of loneliness, but the self-concept principles begin operation. They become anti-male so most males see them as anti-male and begin to treat them in an "anti-" manner. All this further reinforces their beliefs about men and the self-perpetuating, vicious cycle, "snowball" is in full speed down the hill. Her error of judging the entire male population by the "scrote" minority will debilitate (cripple) her the remainder of her life.

B) How many times have you heard someone say, "You can't keep anything nice any more. Everyone just tears it up," when that person has just had something precious destroyed or vandalized. Well, the error in the above sentence is the word "everyone." If you, for example, take pride in the appearance of your home, most of us will take pride in your home and treat it accordingly. But I already know some problem person will drive his car across your yard. And the moment you become paranoid and start seeing all of us as potential lawn destroyers, your life is injured more than anyone else's.

C) The classic example is the woman who lets a man physically abuse her and continues to "go back for more." We've learned much about her in recent years and it relates closely to the points I'm trying to make regarding self-concept and its vast importance. She will most always tell us in the beginning that she continues to go back because she loves her man so much. Her favorite song is most always "Stand By Your Man." But as time goes by in the counseling relationship, truer motives begin to surface in over 90% of the cases.

Could it be that, unbeknownst to herself, she continually goes back for more because she has a need to be beaten? Probably! Sounds unbelievable, doesn't it? But there is much evidence that it is so and it is deeply related to our four principles of self-concept discussed thus far plus the fifth principle soon to be discussed.

First, we find so often, as we do longitudinal studies of habitually abused women, that they have been severely abused either emotionally and/or physically as little girls—usually by a male figure (father, step-father, foster father, grandfather, etc.). So, apparently they have internalized concepts of themselves as women who "deserve" to be beaten.

Closely related, they will most always score high on guilt scales when they take personality tests—proving that they feel deeply that they do not measure up in various ways and thus need to be punished for their "unworthiness" so as to prove to themselves that they are "bad little girls." Evidence of this theory is a typical statement made by these women to their counselor/therapist: "I guess if I'm really honest with myself, I deserved my beating because I really didn't have his supper ready." How sad it is when you realize that she's really serious—that she "deserved" to have her face beaten in due to not performing some trivial task required by her "scrote" husband. I might add that, in my opinion, men who beat women are not even as important to the universe as a piece of manure in the field. The manure performs a much more essential function. And if they are not willing to seek professional help, they would do the world a great favor by committing suicide. The same is true of women who beat upon men or parents who abuse children. Assault of another person's body without his permission (in contact sports we are granting permission) is unforgivable as far as I'm concerned.

The final proof, however, of her unconscious need to be beaten is the most conclusive. We have already established that she has habitually and continually returned to her "beater" in order to become the "beatee." But let's say, for whatever reason, she finally gets away from scrote man. Naturally, enough is enough, right? No more of that life-style, right? Wrong! We are dumbfounded how often she will unconsciously, but assuredly, gravitate toward another man who will again beat upon her body. She just can't seem to help herself. It's just her nature or, in this case, her internalized self-concept.

All of this is a true lesson in self-concept, which leads us to principle #5—and the one most relevant to this book. Obviously, you see yourself as fat; you treat yourself as fat; others treat you as fat; others see you as fat; so you gravitate toward fatness! Not convinced, are you? I don't blame you, so now we must look at Principle #5 of self-concept psychology—AND BY FAR THE MOST IMPORTANT!

5) THE HUMAN ORGANISM WILL CONTINUALLY, DILIGENTLY, AND RELENTLESSLY—BOTH CONSCIOUSLY AND/OR UN-CONSCIOUSLY—WORK TO FULFILL THE INTERNALIZED IMAGE IT HAS OF ITSELF!

The statement you have just read is the single most important statement in this book! In my opinion, it is the single most important sentence that you will read/hear in your lifetime! Please go back and read it again right now. It is the very backbone of this book and the Jerry L. Walke program. Please commit it to memory. Now, we must break it down and analyze it completely because I'm truly convinced the remainder of your life on this earth will now completely revolve and evolve around the above statement.

PSYCHO-CYBERNETICS

You may recognize the term "psycho-cybernetics" because it is the title of a very noted self-help book by Maltz. By the way, I highly recommend this book and have for many years. In my opinion, it is the best over-all self-help book ever written and I've sold many copies for Dr. Maltz. I hope to some-day meet him.

In any event, "psyche" has to do with the mind/brain and "cybernetics" is the study of machines and their relationship to man. What we have come to realize more and more in the past 20 years is that the human brain is literally a computer! Yes, LITERALLY a computer, albeit a highly sophisticated and complex computer—nevertheless, an electrical computer, no more, no less.

As you see, hear, feel, taste, and smell any experience, that sensory manifestation is done through pure electrical, psychic energy. You are a machine, pure and simple. Yes, a very unique one made of flesh and blood. Yet, just an electron, neutron, proton, electrical, chemical machine. Your thoughts, your feelings, your instincts—all electrically computerized. Not theory, fact, though you and many others may not like to hear it. We call ourselves human beings and thus, we are labeled "human beings"—but COSMIC FLESH COMPUTER would be just as accurate a name. Sound cold? Of course not! The entire process which "God" used to evolve your computer over billions of years is both awesome and beautiful. We even understand a great deal of it now.

In any event, everything you were, everything you are, and everything you hope to be (we call this whole package "personality") is simply the way your "computer" (brain) has been programmed by others; how you have pro-grammed it yourself; how you interpret that programming; and, most impor-tant of all, HOW YOU PROGRAM YOUR COMPUTER FROM THIS MOMENT FORWARD!

Your self-concept now? Programmed by others and you. Your feelings? Programmed by others and you. Your goals—or lack of goals? Same! Your moral structure? Absolutely! Your obesity? Yep! Everything! Yes, we can even prove that instinctive behavior can be programmed and re-programmed. I don't have time or space to explain such deep behavior modification, but rest assured it is so. Pavlov proved it long ago with his classic experiments with conditioning dogs.

Obviously, man has not yet been able to even come close to building a computer as sophisticated as his own cranial one. I might add that there is lit-tle doubt in my mind that we will do so within the next 50 years as we learn to understand the human brain thoroughly—if we do not blow humankind from the globe in the meantime. We have learned a great deal about the brain recently and it is reasonable to assume that we will understand it as thoroughly in the near future as we now do the heart.

The beauty of it all is that the human computer (brain) is so intricately intertwined into itself through left-brain, right-brain, cerebral cortex, limbic system, and R-complex that IT IS THE ONLY COMPUTER WHICH CAN PROGRAM AND RE-PROGRAM ITSELF! And that little "universal miracle" is the key to your future. As you learn to program and re-program your psyche, the world becomes yours for the taking. Everything changes—for the better! The statement "you are what you think" is so true that we are just beginning to realize how true it is. I'll show you why soon, but we must first go back and analyze principle #5.

PRINCIPLE #5

THE HUMAN ORGANISM WILL CONTINUALLY, DILIGENTLY, AND RELENTLESSLY—BOTH CONSCIOUSLY AND/OR UNCONSCIOUSLY—WORK TO FULFILL THE INTERNALIZED IMAGE IT HAS OF ITSELF!

Let's scrutinize this statement very carefully. Your future life depends upon this universal truth and it has fantastic implications for you. As mentioned previously, it is the single most important statement your ears will ever hear and that your brain (cranial computer) will ever record.

The statement is reasonably self-explanatory if you read it over a few times, but it does need some additional explanation in order for you to realize its great significance to you and all mankind.

First of all, obviously, the "human organism" means you—but it means you in all your entirety. Your mind, your body, your psychic energy (libido), your emotions, your instincts, your cerebral cortex thinking cells, your conscious mind (that which you can recall), your unconscious mind (that which you can't recall but which, nevertheless, affects your daily behavior greatly), your complete being (called "being alive") on this earth. All the above work together "continually" to fulfill the internalized image you have of yourself. Awesome! But even more awesome is the fact that these dynamic forces not only work continually, but even "diligently and relentlessly" toward self-fulfillment. "Diligently and relentlessly," of course, means that your entire being is working hard and strenuously and unceasingly to move toward the finalized "picture" you have of yourself at any given time. Scary, huh,—especially if that mental image is negative and destructive! Also scary because it can be inverted. That is, whatever direction you are going at any given time reflects an internalized NEED you have to go in that direction. Whew!

But even more frightening when you add the dimension of "unconsciously." As stated above, "unconscious mind" simply refers to those thoughts and experiences we've had through the years that we can't recall. Yet these unknown brain "stowaways" have a great affect upon our behavior patterns at any moment, minute, hour, day, etc. They control us as much (probably more) than do our conscious thoughts.

We may not be able to recall certain material just because the perception isn't strong enough. For example, a person you met only once six years ago. Or we also often can't recall an experience because our psychic energy works against recalling it—usually due to the fact that that experience is negative and threatening to us in some manner. That process is called anti-cathexis (Freud), repression and denial. For example, we may continually forget (repress) a person's name that we've met many times because that person is in some manner (unconsciously, probably) a threat to us. In any event, unconscious factors are a vital force in shaping our daily behavior. Yet, we need not fear unconscious elements. They can usually be controlled and programmed quite readily, also. I'll show you how soon.

So many people fear the unconscious mind and believe that it is some secret compartment in the brain that may contain some unknown psychological monster that may, at any time, escape and do them in—that is, drive them crazy. That is quite doubtful.

It is my belief that is quite easy to tell whether or not you have some thought patterns built around previous negative experiences "lurking" in your unconscious mind. That is, do you display or manifest some form of bizarre behavior. If so, then you probably do have some repressed conflict patterns "lurking." For example, let's say that you are a woman and almost every time you pass a man, the thought immediately pops into your mind that he is going to rape you. Even though you know it's not so, the thought still comes into mind. Let's further say that you find this fixation (hang-up) to be quite burdensome and that it has rendered you distant and incapable of an intimate relationship with a man. Do you have some repressed material "lurking?" Probably! Most would agree your behavior is bizarre. Therefore, some bizarre experience(s) may well have befallen you and bizarre thought patterns emanated from that. Can those patterns be changed? In all probability! Can you change them yourself? Oftentimes!

Finally, let's discuss briefly the term "internalized image." Simple, but a little tricky, too. Tricky because the "internalized" image is usually different from the image we like to admit to ourselves we have. We usually rationalize a positive picture to ourselves and others while we are quite busy (continually and diligently) fulfilling almost the complete opposite image. For example, the athlete who repeatedly says he has a need to win while continually displaying losing type efforts or, more relevant to our case, the person who states over and over that he/she wishes to be slender but continues diligently to work toward obesity.

It is so apparent as you observe humans closely over many years that our external self-concept and internalized (down deep) self-concept are just too often not consistent. Thus, the universal importance of Socrates' classic statement: "KNOW THYSELF." Easily said, but difficult to do. But again, I'll show you how to do so.

EXAMPLES OF PRINCIPLE #5

Let's take a look at some typical examples of this principle at work in our everyday lives:

A) How often you have heard, or made, this statement? "There is no excuse for being dirty—any one can afford soap." Of course, you're right. At least in this country and in the western world, anyone can afford soap. In fact, given a forced choice, you and I would probably beg, borrow, or even steal soap rather than go dirty. Right? So, why are there so many dirty, filthy people?

You know the answer, don't you? Yep, self-concept principle #5! If a person has an internalized image of himself as dirty and unworthy, he'll continually, diligently and relentlessly—both consciously and unconsciously—work to be dirty and unworthy. Buy for him a semi-truck loaded with soap, detergent, paint, shampoo, deodorant, toothpaste, Lysol, ad infinitum—and he'll still be dirty and unworthy. It is his "scorpion" nature—that is, his internalized image. Like I said, it's tricky, because he'll usually state (and believe) that he wants to be clean (remember, all athletes say they want to win). And he'll even become angry if you tell him you think he really wants to be dirty. Can he change? Of course, if he reads this book and takes it seriously—just as you will change if you continue to read and are taking it seriously. But until he gains knowledge into his own conduct, and truly wishes to change, he NEVER will. He's destined to be dirty. Now you see why education is so important.

B) Let's discuss a great example that I've used over the years in my classes: The movie HUSTLER with Paul Newman, Jackie Gleason, and George C. Scott. (I'll probably be paraphrasing in most cases since the movie is 15-20 years old at least).

In the movie, Paul Newman played the role of "FAST EDDIE," a young, talented, brash, cocky pool shooter. Jackie Gleason played "MINNESOTA FATS," the world's champion pool shooter (at least in that movie portrayal, if not in true life), and George C. Scott was carefully developed as a highly streetwise, professional gambler—an expert at psychologically sizing up anyone and everyone, the ultimate "Ph.D." in experience. He "bankrolled" Minnesota Fats and simply followed Fats from town to town collecting his percentage of the winnings and leading the good life.

"Fast Eddie" also followed, carrying his own "stash" since he had no "sugardaddy" (yet) to bankroll him. He repeatedly tried to challenge "The Fat Man" into a match so that he could prove that he was the best in the world—not Fats. Gleason rejected him on the basis that "You ain't got no reputation, kid." But Fast Eddie persisted, all the while beating some very good players while pursuing Fats from city to city. Finally, Fats felt compelled to answer the challenge of the fast rising reputation of Eddie and an extended match of straight pool was agreed upon—for big bucks. George C. Scott, whose money was at stake, perched himself stealthily on a high stool in the background to watch the action. Obviously, his eyes and mind missed nothing.

The match began and it became evident quickly that Eddie was good—darn good. He flitted confidently and cockily around the table, pocketing every conceivable type of shot. He carried a small flask of whiskey from which he took periodic sips in order to make certain he continued to shoot a "loose stick." He built a big lead on Fats, quite bedraggled and "shook" by this time, and taunted "The Fat Man" as he gained big winnings—thousands of dollars. "I thought you 'was' supposed to be good Fat Man," he gloated.

Later, both players agreed to take a break in the action for ten minutes. Gleason, perspiring profusely, with his ever-present carnation wilting, approached George C. Scott and stated something similar to "He's tough, too tough, I can't beat him. He's the best young player I've ever seen. Do you want me to continue? It's your money."

George C., quiet and observant to this point, looked at Fats and said, as only the gravel-voice Scott can, "Oh, yes, Fats, by all means continue, he is a pure loser." In the back of the room, Newman overhead the cut and simply smirked confidently. Fats, meanwhile, gave George C. Scott an "Are you serious" facial expression and went to freshen up, doubt registering all over his face and walk.

The match continued, and Eddie continued to dominate. But you guessed it. Suddenly the shots that Eddie had been making were hanging at the edge of the pocket. And soon he wasn't even coming close. Then he began to press, his confidence waned, and his stick tightened. Fats became confident and Newman now became an easy mark. Fats won back all his previously lost money plus every penny Eddie owned. Eddie was humiliated and his "stash" was gone.

Yes, the whiskey had taken its toll. Newman was by this time drunk and wasted, unable to even focus on the balls, and the "loose stick" had become a shakey stick. He staggered from the poolroom, but stopped at the door to proclaim, "I'm better than you, Fat Man, and would have beaten you IF I hadn't of got drunk." Gleason gave an "I know it, kid" gesture while Scott simply snorted quietly. He knew the kid was a self-destructor—what we call in psychology a high abasement need person. In short, he knew what Eddie's internalized self-concept was and that it was only a matter of time until he relentlessly pursued it.

Newman then drifted from bar to bar "hustling" local players—shooters with far less talent than his own that he'd lure into money games by pretending to be drunk and in possession of little pool-shooting ability. It was only a matter of time until disgruntled red-neck "fish", bitter at being taken, would vent their aggressions upon Eddie. This finally happened when a group of "bad asses" broke both his thumbs.

From this point on, the movie shows Newman "learning his lesson," at least to an extent, and "getting his act together." Toward the conclusion of the flick, Newman, now again somewhat established as a legitimate pool shooter, attends a party at Scott's expansive, expensive home. Newman collars Scott in his den and asks, "How did you know Fats would beat me? Why did you call me a loser?"

Scott eyed him carefully and rasped in his inimitable gravel voice (again paraphrased), "Son, I've watched people like you come and go for years—and you are a loser BECAUSE YOU CONTINUALLY LOOK FOR AN EXCUSE TO LOSE! This statement was the major thrust of the movie and possibly the hardest-hitting statement you or I will ever hear. It has so much to say about self-concept psychology and, more specifically, to weight loss and weight control. Seldom have I met an obsessive-compulsive eater who hasn't developed a highly sophisticated network of "excuses to lose."

But back to the movie and its meaning to principle #5. Newman looked at Scott increduously and said, "C'mon, you know I'm better than Fats and would have beaten him if I hadn't of gotten drunk." And Scott then informed Eddie that that was the entire point. He was playing for the world's championship; an opportunity for wealth, fame, and prestige; a chance to "be somebody." Yet, UNCONSCIOUSLY, his entire "organism" worked continually, diligently, and relentlessly to certainly lose. He possessed an internalized image of himself as losing and simply doggedly fulfilled it.

As mentioned previously, we call it HIGH ABASEMENT NEEDS in the field. Freud called it "too strong of a death instinct." Scott aptly labeled it "continually looking for an excuse to lose." I could discuss examples the remainder of this book if I wanted because high abasement people are usually easy to pick out. But we need discuss only one more example:

C) Yes, foodaholics truly fulfill principle #5. We are at the very heart of self-concept and cybernetics and the intermingling of the two. If you are grossly overweight (fat, obese, etc.), then, with rare exceptions, you are showing yourself—and the world—that you have an internalized image of yourself as fat—or unworthy/guilt-ridden in some manner—and that you are into the diligent pursuit of being fat—or of unworthiness/guilt.

The cycle is a very vicious one which feeds upon itself. To put it bluntly, the fatter you become, the fatter you become! That is, the more you obsessively-compulsively eat; the more you see yourself as obese; and the harder you work toward those ends. Tragic? Sure, and of course most of it is probably unconscious on your part. But still true. And most every diet program I've encountered is a battle in futility because it unwillingly, but continually, reminds you that you are fat. Therefore, no programming—except negative programming—is really taking place in your computer. I'll explain this very soon.

BOTTOM LINE

You are obese because you are programmed obese—either by yourself or others, probably both! Therefore, it is up to you to begin to re-program yourself. Only YOU can do it, though I will help you along the way—at least here in the beginning months. As mentioned previously, you did not get programmed (conditioned) toward "fatness" overnight and you will not recondition yourself toward "slenderness" over night—but it can and will happen. Be patient and gentle with yourself and be patient and cooperative with me. Do not fight against yourself as you have been doing with your "neurotic" foodaholism. Just relax and let it all happen. Your life will soon be changing wonderfully! I'll mention my favorite quote three or four times throughout this book:

THERE ARE NO LEGITIMATE EXCUSES FOR BEING GROSSLY OVERWEIGHT . . . ONLY EXCUSES!

CHAPTER NINE

Let's Begin Programming

I want to make a few points clear from the beginning regarding the re-programming of your cranial computer (brain) as it relates to weight loss:

1) There is more than one method for programming and re-programming. However, they are all similar and I'll be giving you the method I have found simplest (K.I.S.S.—Keep It Simple, Stupid!) and most effective in my work through the years. Most of the great ideas in the history of the world have been elementary, simple ideas, ranging from mathematical equations to compound interest; from flying to sub-dividing land; and from the internal combustion engine to life insurance. Once they are understood, they are simple.

2) As stated in part one of this book, I believe a support person—especially during the first few months—renders your efforts more effective. If the support person is someone you trust, then he/she can even perform your programming periodically. Actually, I recommend it, but only once or twice a week because you must learn to program yourself (auto-programming). Remember what I said earlier—if you don't do it, it won't get done.

THE PARABLE OF BRAD'S TRICYCLE

Before we continue with our tri-lateral programming, permit me to relate a true and relevant story to you to emphasize the importance of the above statement, "If you don't do it, it won't get done."

My son, Brad, is now 21 years old. He has been a high quality son of whom I'm quite proud and he has already accomplished a great deal in his young life. To list here all his achievements would be clearly presumptious, so suffice it to say that his credits academically, athletically, and socially/humanistically would be documented by most people who have known him—not just me as his prejudiced father. At his graduation (from a well regarded high school), a veteran guidance counselor publicly acclaimed him as "The best all-around male graduate from this high school in my many years here."

There were many factors leading to Brad's magnanimous successes and many people could be given credit. But I am convinced that one significant event in Brad's life SYMBOLIZED why he was so achievement oriented and that a major reason he was so autonomous during his first two decades on this earth was because his mother and I continually related to him in the same same manner as we did on this occasion.

It all happened when Brad was a youth of approximately three and one-half years. Like most boys, he had a tricycle, and like most boys, he had already mastered that vehicle to the point at which he could ride it very fast. We had a circular driveway in front of our home and Brad dearly loved to "lickety-split" around that oval, using both the pedals and his feet to propel him in lightning-like fashion.

One Saturday morning he was "doing his thing" and I happened to be observing the whole scenario from the living room picture window. However, the drapes were drawn shut so that he did not know I was watching. As he sped around and around his "race track," he suddenly encountered another situation that most of us experienced as young boys. The tricycle got out of his control and began to tilt past the limits of centrifugal force. His efforts to right it were in vain and he toppled to the blacktop with the trike on top of him. The front wheel turned and instantly caused the handlebars to encircle his chest and entrap him against the pavement. Almost all of us men (and probably most women) can remember when we suffered a similar catastrophe with our tricycle or bicycle.

Now, please keep in mind that my close witness of this event made me realize that Brad was not seriously hurt and was in no danger. His head had not hit anything and his limbs had not bent in any manner, so he at most could only have suffered minor cuts or abrasions. But his reaction was that of a classic "All-American" child.

Because this traumatic event frightened him, he immediately sent out the "fire alarm" to the giant fire engine in the kitchen—his mother. He began to cry loudly and scream "mommy" at the top of his lungs. Verna (his mother) heard the five-alarm plea and also responded in instinctive motherly fashion. She spontaneously yelled my name as she raced from the kitchen, through the dining room, and toward the front door.

However, I intercepted her with a quieting finger to my lips and a halting gesture with my other hand. "He's all right, Verna," I explained, "I saw the whole thing and he's not hurt." Brad's mother hastened to the window and saw him sprawled on the drive with the tricycle on top of him. "Oh, Jerry, he's hurt," she shrieked, and headed full-speed for the door. Uncharacteristically, I grabbed her by the arm and stopped her. "He's O.K. Verna," I assured, "Let's watch what he does next." Verna strained against my taut hand but said nothing because we both had always practiced a fairly consistant philosophy of child-raising.

Well, Brad continued to cry loudly and scream for his "mommy." And mommy continued to look distraught and strain against my restraint. And I continued to console her by guaranteeing his welfare and urging her to wait for phase two of this "emergency."

Soon Brad realized that mother was not coming to lick his wounds and kiss all and make it well. So, indeed he did enter phase two. His fear turned to aggresion (true of all human behavior) and he began to yell ferociously and kick and beat on his tricycle. But this unorganized wrath served no purpose (get the message?) and he remained pinned to the blacktop. Phase three was about to begin. In the meantime, Verna was berating me, "See, Jerry, he can't get up!" and was straining at the bit to rush to Brad's rescue. "Cool it, Verna, let's see what he does next."

Well, finally Brad instinctively realized that unbridled aggression was getting nowhere, so he sent out an even louder alarm for the fire-engine woman. "Mommy!" he repeatedly yelled—at about forty-six decibels. This was more than any mammal mamma can bear, so Verna tried to break my vise-like grip on her biceps. "Just a little longer," I pleaded, and she gave in.

And now came the golden moment. Now Brad internally came to the realization that all of us must reach—and the younger and sooner we comprehend this universal truth, the better. For now, you see, Brad consciously and unconsciously knew that there was no one there to help him. He knew that if the problem was to be solved, he was going to have to solve it. YES, HE KNEW THAT IF IT WAS TO BE DONE, HE HAD TO DO IT! What a great teaching/learning moment this was!

Brad grew quiet and his mental wheels began to turn. And he started using his cerebral cortex (logic) rather than his limbic system (emotions). He twisted, strained, fulcromed, levered, muscled, and crawled from that octopus-like tricycle and soon he was free. And then another wonderful thing occurred. Completely within our line of vision, he hopped to his feet and climbed back upon his tricycle. His face was lit up as though a spotlight had been focused on it as he came directly toward us in his re-newed journey around the driveway. He had solved his own problem; he had controlled his own destiny; he had captained his own ship. Minor occurrence, you say? Well, maybe, but you know better, don't you? What would we have solved if "mommy" had run to his aid? Nothing! What would he have been learning? Absolutely nothing, except that someone would always be there for him in troublesome times.

Well, folks, that's just not the way it is in this cosmos, and unfortunately, many do not learn this universal truth until they're 20, 30, 40 or never. Brad was fortunate that he was learning it (being taught it, though he didn't know it) at 3½.

And the Brad Walke Parable is completely relevant to your weight loss. Sure, I'll teach you how, just as we did Brad. But if it's to be done, you must do it!! I might add here that my next book, almost finished in rough draft manuscript, will be entitled RAISING CHILDREN FOR THE 21ST CENTURY. One of the major points I'll discuss in that book is that one of the glaring weaknesses of American mothers is that they far over-protect, over-control, and over-indulge their children. This is probably just another cause of obsessive-compulsive eating and gross obesity in our children. I am a great believer in Froebel's basic concept that children should learn to grow up under the stars—roughly.

3) Before you ask an obvious question, permit me to answer it. Yes, all this will be a combination of meditation, semi-self-hypnosis, daydreaming, and fantasizing. It is the organization of these that is the key. In essence, you are going to be organizing your daydreams. And don't treat "organized daydreaming" lightly. It will, along with some other techniques, work wonders in your life.

Tri-Lateral Programming

INTRODUCTION

Remember, you and I agreed many pages ago that every facet of my program is essential; that no part of it should be seen as juvenile or "silly;" and that only following ALL instructions will lead to your change from living to eat to eating only to live—that is, the "cure" of your foodaholism. I have studied the 10% failures with whom I've worked, and they've invariably always thought some part of my program either unnecessary or "dumb" (looking for excuses to lose?). Since most of the program has been purposely simplified, there is no reason for you to shirk or omit any part of it unless you truly don't want to become slender. To omit any phase is giving yourself a message.

JUST WHAT
ARE WE ALL ABOUT HERE?

The concepts and principles presented in this chapter are simplified, elementary, and maybe even (to you) juvenile. But please keep in mind that they are based upon deep psychological knowledge. As stated previously, we do not yet understand all there is to understand about that great inner frontier we call the human brain, yet we are learning quickly and we know much more than we did just a short century ago—or even a decade ago.

We are learning more each month about the various lobes of the brain, right brain—left brain, various centers, etc. But one thing we know for certain is that there are three distinct brain areas: the hindbrain, which is probably the oldest and earliest to develop, and housing our basic instinctive needs and desires to survive. Most scientists now refer to the hindbrain as the R-complex. The "R" stands for reptile because not only is our human hindstem structured like all the other higher animals—and performs the exact same functions—but it is even structured like and performs the exact same functions as the reptiles' hindstem. Freud referred to this phase of our personality as the Id. And make no mistake, we are highly instinctive "Id" animals. It's just that we are such highly intelligent animals that we camouflage our instincts better by what we call civilized, refined, sophisticated actions. Our R-complex plays a significant role in over-eating.

The midbrain is usually now labeled the "limbic system," and it houses all our emotions and feelings, which includes all our moral and ethical codes—which is based mainly on emotions. The limbic system, I contend, plays even a greater part in obsessive-compulsive eating and it must be dealt with and re-programmed. By the way, Freud referred to the limbic system as the superego aspect of our personality.

Finally, and most certainly the latest to develop, is the forebrain—or cerebral cortex. It houses our 10-12 billion thinking cells and is where we do all our rational, logical thinking. Any thing you have learned, from tying your shoes to trigonometry and from how to get to Pittsburgh to Latin, was accomplished in the cerebral cortex. Freud labelled this aspect of your personality as the ego.

Obviously, these three distinct brain areas operate simultaneously and in unison (usually), though not without a great deal of conflict in most of us—and usually a great deal of conflict within the obsessive-compulsive foodaholic.

The purpose of everything discussed from this point forward in this book—whether it be simple "stuff" or complicated "stuff"—will be to use the cerebral cortex to re-program and condition the limbic system and thereby permitting BOTH the cerebral cortex and limbic sytem working together to "tame" the R-complex. Can it be done? Of course, we do it all the time! But can you do it? Sure, I'll show you how!

STEP ONE
OF TRI-LATERAL PROGRAMMING

The first step of Tri-lateral Programing is quite simple: RELAX—AS MUCH AS POSSIBLE. No problem here, especially since I added the phrase "as much as possible." I did this because I already know that most of you reading this have some difficulty in relaxing. The very nature of an obsessive-compulsive personality is to have "neurotic-type" daily life patterns which make relaxation difficult. If you are a high-anxiety type person (as I am), deep relaxation is probably almost an impossibility for you—at least at this time.

As you stick with this program, you will learn more and more how to relax. In addition, I'll teach you some techniques of relaxation. The major point to remember right now is that the more relaxed you are the more effective your re-programming will be. Your computer/brain works that way. But even if you have trouble relaxing at first, my principles will work. It'll just take a little longer to see results. Don't sweat it!

Explore yourself a little at this point to discover how you most relax—that is, the physical position you most like to assume. Maybe you like to lie down on a couch or bed, possibly a recliner chair, etc. My personal preference is a very comfortable chair with my feet propped up above my waist, feet crossed, and arms across my chest. Find yours, even if it happens to be standing on your head or lying in a hot tub of water (which I highly recommend).

Then, before performing step #2, I go through some rituals in order to relax myself as much as possible. I call these rituals my D.R.T.—Deep Relaxation Technique—and have found them quite effective with both myself and counselees. Use them if you like. With daily practice, you can learn to ALMOST hypnotize yourself (semi-auto-hypnosis) with these rituals:

A) BODY TIGHTENING

This is nothing new but it works. Start with your toes and tighten them literally as hard as you can for a count of five. Then relax them and concentrate your mind on your toes for a few seconds, feeling the nice tingling sensation that usually follows. Now do exactly the same with the entire foot. Then the calves; then the thighs; the hips; the stomach; chest, arms; hands; neck; and face. Each time, concentrate briefly on that relaxed, tingly body part when you un-flex. Finally, tighten your whole body—from toes to face—at the same time for a count of five. Then relax all and feel yourself sink into your chair/bed/couch with a deeply relaxed feeling. You might wish to repeat the final over-all tightening five or six times. In fact, again I recommend you to do so. Not only are you relaxing more with each un-flexing but you are toning the body with each flex.

B) DEEP BREATHING

After completing the body tightening, I feel very nice—and keep in mind that I am a high anxiety person with a great deal of natural body tension. I have been doing these rituals EVERY DAY for four years and find them cumulatively better. That is, with time I become more and more relaxed. Rome was not built in one day. Deep relaxation is not learned in one day. And eating patterns are not altered in one day.

Now I begin the second phase of my relaxation ritual—one which brings me a very natural "high." I begin a very slow count up to ten—allowing approximately 20-30 seconds between each count. I concentrate on my lungs and breathing and begin by taking BREATHS slightly deeper than normal. I keep my inhalations/exhalations very, very rythmic. This is imporant. With each count upward, I breathe a little deeper until—by the time I've reached "ten"—I'm respirating very deeply. When I'm finished, I'm nearly as high as any alcohol high I've ever experienced (I don't do any drugs). This naturally induced "high" is a wonderful, euphoric high that also becomes better with time and practice.

I'm convinced this "high" has scientific, physiological causes. I'm certain the blood becomes overloaded with oxygen, which naturally soon reaches the brain, and has the same effect as breathing pure oxygen, especially when you are lying down and inactive. It is a great feeling which I have learned to depend upon each day for stress management. And as with the body tightening, I've become better and better with it with the passage of time. Try it. You should check with a physician if you have any reason to believe that you shouldn't hyper-oxygenate in this manner or if you hyper-ventilate for some reason.

C) FREE FALL AND TICK-TOCKING

Now I begin a backward count from ten, concentrating on the ticking of a clock stationed nearby and mentally imagining that I'm either falling (safely) or flying. With each count downward, I imagine myself falling further down or flying higher—but in each case being freer and freer. When I'm finished with these three phases, I'm usually (not always) in a state of almost suspended animation/hybernation/twilight sleep semi-auto-hypnosis. It is a wonderful, relaxed feeling which I've slowly, but surely, learned to self-induce. Again, try it. Now, deeply relaxed, steps #2 and #3 which follow will be more beneficial. Remember, as you learn to relax more and more—and it IS learned—your tri-lateral programming will be more effective. Since you'll be doing it EVERY day, you'll be getting a lot of practice.

RELAXATION RITUALS "FRINGE BENEFITS"

It is no secret to anyone that relaxation—and the accompanying peace of mind—is one of the great gifts one can possess. There is no medication that can produce the therapeutic benefits that come from being freed from the chains of stress and tension. However, due to the complexities of the human brain and nervous system, and due to the built-in stress of life in a modern, scientific, over-populated, mass news media, nuclear world, stress management has become a major problem. With most of us, feelings of complete relaxation are not easy to attain. My program of relaxation rituals, plus the remainder of my self-concept psychology to be presented soon, has produced some additional benefits.

For example, I've had quite a few clients who are students in a registered nursing curriculum. There is almost always great pressure in the R.N. program and students often complain of their problems in taking tests, even though they "know the material." I've had at least four nurses' testimonials that, after completing my program, they've had much more successful experiences in test taking. Some have even overcome mild and moderate panic attacks that they have experienced prior to or during test taking.

I've had at least ten people who've suffered anxiety reactions (a mild type of "nervous breakdown") tell me that my program enabled them to recover more quickly. I've had many athletes state that my techniques enabled them to better handle pressure and, therefore, reach their physical potentials. A young state champion pistol shooter even recently informed me that "I would never had won had it not been for you." I have actually had people tell me that their recurring nightmares have eased after a few months of these simple techniques. Many other examples could be given. Suffice it to say that as you learn to relax, all of life and health usually improves. Momentary feelings of relaxation and peace of mind are very therapeutic. Prolonged periods of same produce a feeling of well-being that leads one to believe that life is truly wonderful and that "I can conquer the world and make it my oyster." You can learn to induce such feelings within your cranial computer. I'll give you additional proven methods of creating excellent peace of mind later.

STEP TWO
OF TRI-LATERAL PROGRAMMING

Step two of Tri-lateral Programming is going to require 20 MINUTES PER DAY—EVERY DAY!!! This is a cheap price to pay for the extensive and beneficial results you'll receive. Just think, ONLY 20 minutes per day, but EVERY DAY!

YOU ARE FOREWARNED!

Since I have been "down the road" and "around the block" many times in conducting my program, I'll warn you right now that this is the major point at which you'll fail. This stage, Step Two, is one of my barometers with clients to discover whether they (you) are truly serious about weight loss-weight control or simply paying "lip-service" while their programmed internalized image of fatness marches onward. Early in this book I informed you that your foodaholism did not develop overnight and it will not be conquered instantaneously. I also stated that I could usually pick my future failures quite early in counseling. Why? Because here at Step Two they will begin to invent every excuse in the book why they won't be able (or weren't able as the first few weeks went by) to spend 20 minutes per day—EVERY DAY! They are, by their actions, already telling me and themselves that they are doomed to a life of burdensome obesity.

I said EVERY DAY! Not taking a day off periodically. Every day, not taking weekends off—or holidays. EVERY DAY. It will "cost" you 20 minutes per day—EVERY DAY—until you reach your target weight. If you aren't willing to pay this price, then don't try to convince yourself, or me, that you are sincere. If you fail in my program, this will probably be the place. But if you spend 20 minutes daily doing specifically what is instructed, you will almost certainly be successful.

THE EXCUSES

I've heard them all—many more times than once, so spare me.

A) The favorite. "I simply don't have time to take 20 minutes EVERY DAY. You just don't know how busy my day is with work, school, the children, etc." Well, I've heard that "I don't have time" rationalization millions of times. And it's just that—pure "cop-out" rationalization. All humans make time for their top priorities. Apparently, weight loss and the conquest of foodaholism is not one of yours. Quit wasting your time reading this book and thank you for buying it. I just made a few bucks off you, though I'll probably give the money to either charity or I.R.S.

Whenever anyone plays the "I don't have time" game with me, I play an interesting little game with them in return. I simply change the subject, yet make certain that the conversation continues. After a while, I'll mention some outstanding TV show I saw recently. Did they happen to see it? "Oh, yes, wasn't that good!" Later I throw in a ballgame or sitcom I really enjoyed. Yes, they saw that, too. I mention an outstanding movie or musical concert. Yep, they attended. A soap opera? They watch it fairly often or regularly. Various restaurants or night spots. "Oh, I've been there!" Like I said, we make time for that which we want to make time. I'm not stupid. I may have been born in the morning—but not YESTERDAY morning.

B) "I forgot a couple of times last week."

"Oh, you forgot?"

"Yes."

"Don't insult my intelligence, fellow human being. We 'conveniently' forget what we want to forget. It's called anti-cathexis, denial, repression, whatever. Your psychic energy works against you recalling that which is a threat to you in some manner."

"No, Dr. Walke, I just forgot. Don't try to psychoanalyze me and get Freudian with me."

"O.K., one question. Did you forget to eat last week, also? Nope, you didn't. Get the message? If you keep forgetting to do your 20 minutes, quit wasting your time with my program. I love you as a fellow struggling person, and I thank you for the approximately $2.00 I profitted from selling you this book, but go no further. Did you forget to put your clothes on today? Did you forget your car on the freeway? Did you forget to take down your pants while urinating? No, of course not. And this 20 minutes, if you're truly genuine in your desire to change, is absolutely as essential as all those things. Our entire program is built on it. The veritable BACKBONE of our success is: 20 minutes per day—EVERY DAY! Do you understand? It is assignment #8."

C) "Doing it every day is silly/dumb/stupid/unnecessary." We've already covered that. Nothing recommended here is silly, dumb, stupid or unnecessary. If you think so (and I'm very serious), prepare to wallow in your obesity forever and prepare your will for an extra large coffin and a very big cemetery lot. My own father believed many of my principles "silly." Yet, I have no doubts that he would be alive today (and healthy) had he read this book many years ago and not considered it "silly." Therefore, I'm not interested in hearing your "silly' excuses. By the way, my dad probably would not have heeded my advice in this book. Isn't it amazing how seldom fathers listen to the ideas of their sons and vice versa? We call that the Oedipus Complex in psychology, but then that's another topic for another book.

IMPLEMENTATION OF YOUR
20 MINUTES PER DAY—EVERY DAY

Invariably, I get the questions of when, where, and why? The "Why" has already been addressed. We are "hanging our hat" on 20 minutes per day—every day because your programming and re-programming will take place here. It is EVERYTHING! My program is negated entirely without the 20 minutes per day.

WHERE?

The more isolated and quieter, the better. Obviously, if you can get off to yourself where it is very, very quiet, then cranial computer programming will take place much more deeply. However, you can still accomplish "change" with some distraction—so long as the distraction isn't completely distracting. A library is fine. Your living room is O.K.—unless your spouse and children are going BERSERK! Go to the car (not while driving of course). Go into your bedroom and shut the door. Take a walk and lean against a tree. If your spouse and children will not let you have 20 minutes of your own completely on your own per day, then it's time you became firm. Time to yourself is your constitutional right. Tell them I said so. Gee, ain't it "funny" how children and spouses too often come to believe that they OWN you. Mother-in-laws tend to follow this ownership syndrome, too.

WHEN?

The time of day that you utilize your 20 minutes is relatively important, in my opinion. Any time you choose to do your 20 minutes is better than nothing, of course, but it is best if you DON'T do it right before going to bed at night or right after getting up in the morning. Take a "time out" period to enjoy your 20 minutes sometime during your active, waking day—whether it be at 10:00 A.M., Noon, 4:00 P.M., etc.

There are definite reasons for this. One, it is psychologically symbolic that you are very serious in your pursuit of a new, internalized self-concept. Two, it is relaxation you need during a hectic day. As mentioned earlier, you will progressively learn to relax more and more with practice and this relaxation is essential in dealing with "neurotic" obsessive-compulsive eating. In fact, non-relaxation is usually one of the major characteristics of foodaholics. Three, there might be a tendency for you to doze off or at least have your mind wander from the task at hand (soon to be discussed) if you use your 20 minutes while in bed.

That reminds me of another excuse I sometimes get from clients or readers. They tell me that they relax so much that they go to sleep and, therefore, do not use their 20 minutes properly. Whenever I encounter these persons, I usually immediately confront them and question their sincerity in the program and their true desire to change. This is simply just another (unconscious probably) excuse to lose. That would be like telling me "I am starving to death because I keep falling asleep at every meal;" or "I am thirsting to death because I keep falling to sleep with every glass of water;" or "I can't drive a car because I keep falling asleep and running off the road." Then you had best visit a local psychologist and/or your physician for narcolepsy. The truth is that we stay awake during the PRIORITY activities of our daily lives. Do you fall asleep during sex, too? If so, you are truly beyond hope.

STEP THREE
OF TRI-LATERAL PROGRAMMING

CREATIVE MENTAL IMAGERY
OR "ORGANIZED DAYDREAMING"

The tough part is over—now for the fun. You read correctly. If you fail, it will probably be your failure to relax as much as possible 20 minutes per day—EVERY DAY, not in this third phase. This, Step Three, will be where we get the work done, of course. It is where we will accomplish the all-important programming and re-programming. But, surprisingly, it is the easiest part. It's all down hill from here—even pure fun—if done correctly.

PRINCIPLE #3

MENTALLY PICTURE THE END RESULT
AT ALL TIMES AND NOT THE PROCESS

Yes, you see, you will be spending your 20 minutes per day—EVERY DAY (tired of hearing that?)—creatively mentally picturing the end result and not the process. It is easy; it is enjoyable; and the outcomes will be so unbelievable that they will "knock your socks off"—and fat, also. But there are definite skills involved in this "end result" imagery and we'll soon learn them.

WHAT NOT TO DO?

You are going to spend your 20 minutes every day simply getting into a relaxed position, closing your eyes, and repeating to yourself such thoughts as: "I am not going to over-eat today;" "I am not going to eat fattening foods today;" "I am going to lose weight;" "I won't eat sweets today;" "I'm sick of my clothes not fitting properly;" "No more desserts;" etc. Do all those (and hundreds of others) statements sound familiar? Others might include "I'm starting my diet tomorrow;" "I'm going to be a vegetarian;" "I'll starve myself;" "I'll start a high protein diet;" "I'm going to eat a light lunch;" etc. It is astounding how many weight-loss programs recommend the above statements—either knowingly or unknowingly.

You are going to repeatedly think those thoughts for 20 minutes, RIGHT? WRONG!! That is the worst thing you can do. That is EXACTLY why most weight programs fail. Such behavior is self-defeating because you are only reminding yourself over and over that you are fat, that you are hungry, and that you are a foodaholic. It is all NEGATIVE PROGRAMMING which gives you an internalized self-image of being obese. Therefore, guess what you—as a human organism—will continually, diligently and relentlessly, consciously and/or unconsciously, work toward? You guessed it. Being fat! You absolutely do NOT spend your 20 minutes in this manner. In fact, all the above statements should NOT be a part of your thoughts at anytime during your waking day. Put aside that jargon forever. It has no place in the new MINDSET that we will be developing. I urge you (beg, if I must) to at least refrain from those statements in your conscious mind at this time. We'll soon take care of the more important unconscious mind. Such thoughts serve absolutely no purpose except destructive ones. They operate only in the realm of will-power and self-discipline and, as already stated, that is not sufficient.

THE COUP DE GRACE

Now for the moment of truth—the fun part. The negative approach above represented the PROCESS. What we're after in your creative mental imagery (organized daydreaming) is the END RESULT. The process is the worst thing you can do with your 20 minutes.

First, keep in mind that the greatest freedom in the cosmos is within your head—that is, the freedom you have to think absolutely anything you want to think. The sky is the limit! Great thinkers think many and great thoughts. They think creative thoughts, often outlandish thoughts. You can think any darn thought you choose. These thoughts are yours and no one else's. They are the most intimate and personal possession you have. So you can spend your 20 minutes in picturing your END RESULT as elegantly and outlandishly as you wish. The more "far out," the better, because you have a lot of programming to do. You've certainly had years of negative programming so we have much to overcome. And that negative programming was just as "outlandish" as any far out positive imagery you can create. But I'll soon show you how!

MY IMAGERY

I'll now share with you my most intimate thoughts in order to show you how it's done. I'll give you examples of how I've spent my 20 minutes the past few years. And lest you laugh at me at times, keep in mind that I wouldn't have to share them because they are mine—just as yours are yours. But I'll "model" them before you so you get an idea of how it's done. Then you can create your own favorite fantasies. Just like Disneyland. But I assure you that what you're doing isn't Mickey Mouse—not if done EVERY DAY on an organized basis.

You should first know that when I began my creative mental imagery I weighed 292 lbs.; wore size 46 pants (which were too tight); and extra, extra large shirts and sweaters—sometimes called tents. You should also know that my target weight was 180, size 32 pants, and medium size shirts. Finally, you might as well also know my little secret: For my tastes in women, there has never been a more beautiful woman—or sexier woman—live on this earth than Natalie Wood. In fact, my fantasies to possess her have been so strong that I didn't even realize until a few years ago that most every woman I've dated since high school; the woman to whom I was married for 24 years; and the woman whom I now love ALL have closely fit the "Natalie Wood prototype." So does the woman I chose to type the manuscript of this book. Ha, I've resented and envied Robert Wagner for many, many years! O.K., now we're ready. I get in my relaxed position, perform a few of my learned relaxation techniques to induce a state of semi-self-hypnosis, and "away we go" for 20 minutes (laugh if you like or must):

A) Mental picture one—my favorite over the years. Roll 'em! There I am walking down the main street of Portsmouth, Ohio. I have on size 32 jeans (always picture the actual size on the label) and a tight medium size short-sleeve, blue T-shirt and cowboy boots. I am slim and trim, lean and mean, cool and cruel (ha).

Three of my students, two women and a male (always picture names and faces) are approaching me. They are talking to each other and I can overhear their conversation:

Woman #1: "There's Dr. Walke, I think he's the sexiest man I've ever seen. Wonder how he got to be built so well."

Man: "I can honestly say he's got the body of a 20 year old. He's unbelievable."

Woman #2: "Look at him, not an ounce of fat on his body, big shoulders and chest, slender hips, hard stomach, what a Hunk! (Keep in mind that I was doing all this while extremely obese).

Keep the above conversation going as long as you like. Enjoy yourself mentally and emotionally. "Get your rocks off!" Might as well because you're doing the exact same thing when you're eating—releasing emotional and sexual energies (libido).

I continue up the street. What's that crowd doing across the street? Looks like reporters and photographers. They are gathered around someone. My God, that's Natalie Wood (her tragic death did not stop my fantasy, "I love you Ms. Wood—wherever you are!") She's stunning. She is wearing a black mini-skirt, black hose, red high heels and a red and black low-cut shirt. In short, the entire outfit is not much more than a wide belt (ha!) and body parts are hanging out all over Chillicothe Street. She has a black Tam hat sitting jauntily sidewise on her head. Flat-out awesome! Good gracious, she has spotted me and is crossing the street toward me. I am frozen. The most beautiful sight my eyes have ever beheld! Makes the Bavarian Alps look like a trash dump. (Note: You tell me how I could ever over-eat for the next week after I'm completely finished with this fantasy. And though I make that statement half tongue-in-cheek, you'll see later that that is precisely what starts happening. I label it "mysterious thinking" and we'll discuss it in great detail). If I held her right now, I'd have everything stacked against me. That's a joke, son!

She IS coming to talk with me. I'm nervous, but confident, Robert Wagner should be so lucky as to look like me. (Wonder if he'd like to have a gladiatorial fight to the finish with maiden Natalie as the prize)?

Natalie speaks as her beautiful brown eyes capture me and draw me into her. "Aren't you Jerry Walke? I've heard so much about your teaching and writing, how sexy and slender you are, and how much you talk of me. Would you have lunch with me at the Ramada Inn? It would be a thrill just to be seen with you, Dr. Walke."

I cannot speak for a few moments. I am awed. Would I have lunch with her at the Ramada? Does a hobby horse have a wooden penis? Are Dolly Parton's feet in the shade?

"I'd be very flattered and pleased, beautiful woman," I finally answer with class and cool, "May I meet you there in an hour?"

"Yes, she replies, "But please do not stand me up. I want so much to know you better."

She turns and walks away and I watch every graceful move of her slender, tapered legs and hips. She glances over her shoulder and winks at me. My entire body tingles with a "magic feeling" but it is a slender, firm body which is undergoing this euphoria, not a fat, roly-poly one. I think to myself as I watch her how wonderful it is to be slender and lean. People with no pride in their appearance do not attract the Natalie Wood's of this world very often.

I immediately head for Portsmouth's best mens' store. There I am walking into the front door and the clerk approaches. "I'd like a nice pair of brown slacks, size 34 please."

"Are you sure you don't want size 32, sir?" He answers, "Those jeans you have on are cut small and they even look a bit loose."

"No thank you, I take size 34."

"As you wish," he said dryly and soon brings me size 34. I go into the dressing room, put them on and, you guessed it, too large.

I walked out sheepishly and tell the clerk "You were right, I do need 32's." He gloatingly retrieves me the correct size, but his gloatiness sure as heck doesn't bother me. I also purchase a medium white sweater and brown suspenders, with a gold choker around my neck, with the V-neck sweater, and the suspenders, I step in front of the mirror. I'm ready for Natalie Wood. Damn, eat your heart out Burt Reynolds, Tom Selleck, Robert Redford, and Paul Newman! Pure sex! (Keep in mind that I'll be discussing the importance of non-vanity soon. This is only a fantasy. But make no mistake a powerful re-programming fantasy. Keep reading).

The male clerk asks, "May I ask, sir, how old are you?"

"Forty-six," I answer truthfully.

"I don't know what your diet and work-out program is," he says sincerely, "But you are the best-built man we've ever had in this shop. To show my genuiness, would you like to model clothes for us?"

I thank him and walk toward the Ramada. The woman I love awaits. (Out of respect for Natalie Wood's death and the feelings of Mr. Wagner, I will not relate the remainder of this detailed fantasy in this book—but rest assured it's a "doozy." Most important, I am continually picturing myself as slender).

B) There I am in the racquetball court, ready to play a young, hard "turk" in the state finals. The crowd is large and excited. The 46 year old veteran versus the lightening-quick, superbly conditioned youth. The old bull against the young bull and youth will surely triumph, right? We'll see about that. Fooling around with the "Walke-man" is about like fooling with Mother Nature and tugging on Superman's cape. I enter the court. Tight, grey shorts, size 32, and blue muscle shirt with white letters emblazoned on the front, "World Class Racquetball—Touring Pro." The fans who have not seen me previously gasp and begin whispering to each other. A young boy says to his father, "Dad, I thought you said he was an old man. He's built better than the young guy."

"I see that, son, he doesn't have ANY extra tissue. Wow, look at the solidness of his arms, shoulders, and legs—and his hard, flat stomach."

Two beautiful young women are also conversing quietly. "Did you say Dr. Walke is single? I'd like to meet him. He is SOMETHING else!" (This fantasy, conducted EVERY DAY, will soon produce some amazing results for me).

"I dream of men like him," says the other, "and his grey hair makes him even sexier. You can tell that he takes great pride in his appearance but that he's not vain or macho about it. There aren't many men around like him." Sometimes I'll go through the entire crowd, picturing SPECIFIC people each time and their SPECIFIC statements.

I have literally hundreds of fantasies like the two above that I've developed over the past four years. You CREATE your own. Never feel guilty about your own thoughts so long as they are positive, progressive, and constructive. Enjoy yourself. The "further out" the thoughts, the better for your programming. By the way, I forgot to mention that in the racquetball imagery, I obviously defeat the young turk quite handily.

You may be thinking at this point that you (or I) can never be as good looking as Morgan Fairchild, Cheryl Tiegs, Burt Reynolds or Tom Selleck. That is not the issue here. The issue is that you take pride in looking as wholesome and beautiful as is humanly possible within your physical limitations. That is continually the ultimate goal—and the only goal! We'll discuss this more later.

YOUR "PARTNER"—IF YOU HAVE ONE

It was discussed early in this book that, admittedly, this entire program is even more effective if you have either a trained counselor and/or friend who can serve as an influential "positive re-inforcer"—especially during the early months. There is no question that another human who likes you and cares for you in an empathetic manner is a great "gift." If you have this partner, it is very beneficial for him/her—during your tri-lateral programming—to induce your relaxation through a steady, calming voice and then to articulate your fantasies (which you have prepared for him in advance) while you are in your relaxed state. I highly recommend this "teamwork," but do not think it should be continued too long. You do not want to develop a dependent relationship.

Does all this constitute hypnosis? In a way possibly, but not really. At most, all the tri-laterial programming, whether alone or with partner, represents a type of semi-hypnosis or semi-auto-hypnosis—while also constituting a form of meditation. I say this because hypnosis is largely misunderstood by most laymen and is therefore a mysterious phenomenon which either awes them or scares them. HYPNOSIS IS AT THE SAME TIME BOTH UNDERRATED AND OVERRATED BY THE AVERAGE MAN IN THE STREET. Doubletalk? Let me explain.

Hypnosis is simply an induced state of deep relaxation, deep "twilight sleep" in which the subject's mind is kind of turned over to or "loaned" to the hypnotist. And in this state, the mind is very susceptible to both probing (examination) and suggestion (programming).

Hypnosis is overrated because may people are frightened that hypnotists have some special powers to control people against their will and that hypnotists are some kind of "shrink"/"witch doctor"/"voodoo" person who can condition their brains to any type of behavior. Actually, anyone can learn easily to hypnotize any other person who will permit (trust) the hypnotist to induce this state. It has been written that only about one of five persons is even capable of somnubulism (a term often used for a very deep hypnotic trance). I disagree. It is my opinion that almost anyone is capable of a somnubulistic state IF they meet a person they truly trust—and IF they practice. It is true that you can't be hypnotized if you don't wish to be (with one exception) and that under hypnosis you will not do anything against your moral and ethical will. However, this becomes "tricky" because we don't always know what our TRUE WILL is—unconsciously. For example, a woman might emphatically state that she would not do a strip tease in public but "down deep" have a desire to do so. Therefore, a show business hypnotist might suggest to her that she do a strip while under hypnotic trance in a Las Vegas night club and her husband and friends might be quite shocked when she begins to do it. It's a more intense version of some of the strange things we say and do under the influence of alcohol and other drugs (which I call "truth serum"—but then that is another story for another day).

Hypnosis is UNDERRATED because of the factors we've discussed throughout this book—that is, the fantastic power of the mind (brain) to control the body and our entire lifestyles and the importance of how the brain (computer) is programmed. Hypnosis and semi-auto-hypnosis are fantastic instruments. This is what I've been trying to tell you from the beginning. They can render some startling effects.

For example, hypnosis is used by many dentists and some of their results are nothing short of mindboggling. Patients in deep hypnotic trances feel no pain without anesthesia or painkiller of any type except the suggestion or command of the doctor. The implications of this are staggering.

The hypnotist's voice, suggestions, and command simply becomes your own. Therefore, if he tells you that you can't raise your arm, then no matter how hard you try, you can't raise your arm because it's yourself telling yourself that you can't raise your arm. We know that if your brain truly believes you can't raise your arm, then it can't be done. This is the entire basis of a neurosis we call conversion hysteria in which sufferers experience blindness, numbness, deafness and paralysis with absolutely NOTHING organically wrong with the afflicted organ or limb. Whew. Talk about mind over matter (body)!

So, do you think if you're told under hypnosis that, at any given time, you are not hungry—then you won't feel hunger pangs? You had best believe it. However, the above is not the thrust of my program and, quite frankly, I don't care for that approach. Again, it only produces, at most, temporary results—and does not change the attitudes and personality behavior patterns so essential to lasting change of lifestyle and the accompanying improvement of quality of life. Nothing permanently positive is gained by turning your life over to others. Remember, if you don't do it, it won't get done!

Our goal in this book is to re-program you to an image of slenderness—knowing that you then will work continually, diligently, and relentlessly to fulfill that image. And the major point is that the technique I have just taught you—somewhere between meditation and semi-auto-hypnosis—is a great programmer and re-programmer, as you practice! Do it daily as though your life depended on it—because it does, either literally or at least psychologically/emotionally.

CASSETTE TAPES

Friends and clients have urged me to cut cassette tapes of my various relaxation techniques and creative mental imageries. To be honest, I haven't done so yet because of procrastination and the time being consumed writing this book. But I plan to in the near future. However, I'll give you a tip to save you money. You can cut your own tape—either of your own voice or your partner's if you have one. Just make certain that you talk in a smooth, even, calming—but firm—voice and go to it. Put your favorite relaxation techniques (body tightening, floating, deep breathing, flying, etc.) and your favorite creative mental imageries on the tape and play it to yourself for 20 minutes on whatever days possible. You may well find that, in your case, the spoken word creates better images (programming) than your own thoughts. It is not unusual for this to be the case.

By the way, in case you actually enter an in-depth hypnotic sleep, wonderful! So many persons fear that they may not "come out of it" if the tapes would break or the command to "awaken" was not presented in some manner. Not true! Just as with a nap, you would soon "awaken" on your own if a hypnotist left your presence—or in this case, if the tape broke or electric failed. In fact, you would probably be aware of the defect almost immediately, according to the depth of your relaxed state.

CONCLUSION

The three stages of tri-lateral programming detailed in this chapter are

EVERYTHING to my program. They must be practiced DAILY until you reach your target weight and have re-programmed yourself away from obsessive-compulsive eating. Tri-lateral programming has worked for hundreds of my clients and it will work for you—if you practice it faithfully. Get started now! Wait until you see what happens. I'll show you soon. "Mysterious" thinking and actions will soon begin to enrich your daily life.

CHAPTER TEN

"Mysterious Thinking"

Now I'll explain a phenomenon that is going to happen to you that you won't believe until it begins to occur in your life—and it most certainly will IF you do your 20 minutes daily—EVERY DAY! This phenomenon has begun in some of my clients within the first two weeks, in others it has taken up to three months. The average is about six weeks—but you can "guarandam-tee" yourself it will take place. So, get ready for it. I have labeled it "MYSTERIOUS THINKING" and if I don't explain it to you, it would "scare you half-to-death" (in a positive way) when it begins. You will not believe how much you're going to enjoy it—because now the unadulterated fun begins.

Actually, "mysterious thinking" is self-concept principle #5 in action and actively at work—"The Human Organism (YOU) WILL CONTINUALLY DILIGENTLY, AND RELENTLESSLY, BOTH CONSCIOUSLY AND UNCONSCIOUSLY, WORK TO FULFILL THE INTERNALIZED IMAGE IT HAS OF ITSELF. Well, you will soon be experiencing it and it will "blow your mind." And it will never stop so long as you continue your 20 minute technique. My "mysterious thinking" has been dynamic and ongoing for almost four years now and it's difficult to describe the results and feelings it has brought me—including the very writing of this book, which I've had in mind for years but accomplished nothing towards its publication. MY LIFE IS NOW SO CHALLENGING BECAUSE OF "MYSTERIOUS THINKING!" I WOULD HAVE GIVEN ANYTHING IF SOMEONE WOULD HAVE TAUGHT ME WHEN I WAS YOUNGER WHAT I'M NOW TEACHING YOU. NO PRICE WOULD HAVE BEEN TOO HIGH FOR THIS BOOK. And just in case your definition of success is monetary, let me say that I would easily be a millionaire by now. Let me explain how my mysterious thinking took place since I have no idea the direction yours might take. But, before I begin, let me say that there is one more assignment (which I'll discuss after this section) which combines with tri-lateral programming to produce this "mysterious thinking." You must fit the ENTIRE package together.

I began my own program approximately four years ago. Though I was practicing weight counseling prior to that time, I was a classic example of "Physician, heal thyself!" and "Not practicing what I preached." Actually, this often happens to doctors, psychiatrists, psychologists, and counselors because of 1) working with others and forgetting self; 2) being "too close to the forest to see the trees"—that is, the difficulty of self-confrontation; and 3) the emotional problems we often encounter simply by constantly dealing with the emotional problems of others. You'd be surprised how easy it is to fall into that trap—probably one of the reasons that the suicide rate is quite high in these professions, and why so many lay people state "I wouldn't go to him. He has more problems than me. He's weird!" I remind you that 15 years ago, when I was doing therapeutic counseling work for mental health clinics, I have documentation that I was improving the quality of many peoples' lives at a time when I was "hurting" most—and was seriously considering taking my own life! That, too, is another story for another day. So let me further elaborate on my wonderful "mysterious thinking" experiences.

My very first "mysterious thinking" encounter was baffling even to me. I have always detested jogging, joggers, and the jogging craze. But my boss, Dr. Scott Come, and some of his colleague college administrators, are really "into" the jogging scene. I had watched their masochistic rituals for years and wanted no part of it. "Hell, they're crazy," I'd think, and I would rather be fat and/or die of a heart attack than participate in such nonsense. Well, after about six weeks of my 20 minute creative mental imagery (and the next technique I'll show you), one day I was in Scotty's office and he was reading a jogging magazine. I stated to him that I didn't realize there was a periodical dedicated to jogging. He answered that there were even more than one and said that he was looking at a new type of jogging shoe and how important proper shoes were. I then said that I hadn't realized that there were special shoes and that I guessed I didn't know much about the field. I could have added that furthermore, I didn't give a darn to know more about the field.

He shoved the magazine into my hand, stated that I was welcome to read it, and I was soon on my way to my office with this "document of punishment" in hand. Arriving at my office, I slapped my own face (literally) and said to myself, "Self, have you gone mad?" and placed that God-awful magazine on my file cabinet with 15 other things I should have read but knew I never would. Good-bye and good riddance to the jogging syndrome. "I must have had a little episode of schizophrenia for a moment," I thought.

Of course, I continued my daily tri-lateral programming. One week later, I found myself sorting out that jogging magazine and then discovering, to my astonishment, that I was leafing through it and even reading a little of that gobbledygook. "Good Lord, what am I doing this for," I introspected. I slapped my face firmly again—thinking all the while that "Oh well, reading doesn't hurt. Heck, I might learn something." And so I kept on reading—and looking at shoe ads and jogging suit ads, etc. Those crazy "nuts" have the field down to a darn science, I discovered. Well, not for me, thank you!

One week later, still continuing my daily 20 minutes (as I still do four years later—I'll tell you about its present state soon), I'm walking by Larry Moore's sporting goods store here in Portsmouth, Ohio. Larry is a longstanding friend of mine, by the way, and a highly reputable businessman. In his show window is a pair of jogging shoes and a complete jogging outfit. My body turned into that store, so help me, as though a huge magnet was drawing me. I performed my face-slapping ritual and rationalized that I was just going in to see my friend, Larry—but I knew better.

Next thing I knew, I'd gotten my Visa card out and purchased the entire works. $110.00, and I almost never buy clothes or anything for myself—haven't for years. Now I'm certain that "I've done gone and blew a gasket" (I love to talk hillbilly). I walk out with that large sack of clothes knowing darn well I'll never use those "garments of ignorance." A complete waste of money.

You guessed it. One week later, I've got that doggone monkey suit on and am walking out the front door to jog a little around the neighborhood. What on earth am I doing, pray tell? Well, I went one block and was completely exhausted. I'm serious! I was ashamed and guilt-ridden at how far my 292 pounds of "lard-ass" had gotten out of shape (atrophied and deteriorated). I walked back that one block, tore off those clothes, and fell into my velour chair to simply grow old and die. As usual, I began to check the television listings for "Hogan's Heroes" and "Taxi."

But, lo' and behold, next day I donned those duds again, hauled my aching butt out the front door, and went two blocks—purely on pride and self-discipline—hating every step. It was pure torture and I swore that my exercise days were over. The next day, further. And the next, and next, and the next—weeks turning into months, months into years. Torturous, but a great feeling when finished, and the fat slowly but surely began to disappear. Now I can jog 14 miles any time I wish—and do I feel super. If I die of a heart attack at this moment, it was all worthwhile, because I was dying anyway.

The important thing to note here is that I still dread and detest jogging. That shows the power of self-concept and the dogged, diligence of our organismal, programmed computer because jogging is now a part of my lifestyle—no longer SELF-DISCIPLINE!

As mentioned earlier, I now jog only a few times per week because my "mysterious thinking" has EVOLVED and led me to a complete exercise program more to my liking and one to reach my goals. That's why I instructed you earlier not to concern yourself in the beginning about a specific program. Your "computer" will handle it for you in a natural manner. Just do your 20 minutes DAILY!

Wait until you hear about "mysterious thinking" #2. To this day, I cannot completely believe it. It was (and is) even more absurd than #1. Pure insanity for certain this time!

I had a beautiful young nursing student in my class named Angela Yvonne Whitt. I knew that "Angee" was a Seventh Day Adventist and a complete (almost) vegetarian. By the way, for your information, I later fell in love with this woman, though I didn't mean to, and hesitantly and painfully ended a 24-year marriage to a very good woman in order to be with Angee. Though I have often been accused of keeping company with my young students over the years, it was not true. It's still difficult to believe that it all happened and, quite frankly, I think it was also all part of MY "mysterious thinking." Though my ex-wife is a tremendous woman; and I could never say anything negative about her; and even though I feel minor guilt over ending my marriage and the hurt it caused within my family—I'm still happier than anytime in my lifetime. "I can't be right for someone else if I'm not right for me"—and the same is true of you! Go to the bank on that statement. It also is at the very heart of self-concept psychology. Even Christ knew that I can't love others if I don't love myself—and neither can you, no matter how much you claim you can.

But back to Angee and vegetarianism and "mysterious thinking." Keep in mind that my entire adult life had been spent as a foodaholic who enjoyed literally all cuisines—American meat and potatoes, bread and butter, bacon and eggs, grease and cholesterol, junk food and more junk food; Italian pizza, lasagna, spaghetti, etc.; Chinese; Polynesian; Japanese; German bratwurst, hard rolls, and kraut; Mexican, from chili to tacos and burritos to enchiladas; French crepes, croissants, and pastries; seafood from oysters to shrimp; from french fried shrimp to fried fish and from crabmeat to scallops; Hungarian; Colonel Sanders; sweets and candies of all types; McDonald's; and whatever. In short, you name it, I ate it—and in great quantities. You may think I'm lying or exaggerating, but many times I went into a restaurant and "showed off" by ordering the entire right side or left side of the menu. My bill might range from $85.00 to $200.00 but I, and whomever were my guests, had a fantastic "pig-out." Friends thought I was flaunting my money. Little did they realize that it was simply the food I was after. The money meant nothing. I was absurdly ravenous most of the time—like most of you are now. Looking back now, the whole scene was 20 years of embarrassment and humiliation.

If you would have told me during those years that I would now be almost a complete vegetarian—and enjoying it—I would have called you a flat-out liar and would have contemplated suicide. I told you my program is potent—because I am now almost a complete vegetarian, and enjoying it immensely. What do you think of that? Here's how my vegetarianism evolved:

Naturally, I was faithfully performing my daily 20 minutes tri-lateral programming (semi-auto-hypnosis) and found that I was quickly becoming better and better at doing so. I discovered the technique that I have already recommended to you—the picturing of specific (very specific) details in your creative mental imagery (organized fantasizing or daydreaming) which soon leads in many cases to a perceptual phenomenon I call "movies or videos on the back of your eyelids."

I had already begun my dreaded—but MYSTERIOUSLY persistent—jogging and evolving a complete exercise program. As mentioned previously, I knew that Angee Whitt—then simply a friend and nursing student—was a Seventh Day Adventist and almost a complete vegetarian. One day I found myself asking her if she had any literature on vegetarianism. To myself, psychologically, I again "slapped my face" and scolded myself for asking. "Where in the heck did those words come from, Jerry?" I was already slowly losing weight and was not about to give up my favorite cuisines—which meant about everything. I had already cut back on portions of all food and, as I said, was shedding pounds. That was sufficient, I rationalized. I certainly don't need to become a vegetarian. Vegetarianism, I thought, is just for nature freaks, liberals and gays.

In any event, Angee said that she not only had presented vegetarian diets and lifestyles to various seminars, but also documented various social, political, and ethical/moral reasons for a concerned, humanistic person to become vegetarian or at least near-vegetarian. A few days later she gave me a book to read regarding vegetarianism and, as with the jogging book previously, I relegated it to my "maybe I'll read it someday" filing cabinet.

But by this time I was vastly underestimating (as you are and will) the power of "mysterious thinking" because I began reading it that VERY evening and found it profound and intriguing. My unconscious organism was again at work fulfilling the new image I was developing (programming) into myself. But I still didn't realize how potent the programming can be. I only knew that, while impressed, I could NEVER give up my life-long favorite meats, starches, gravies, etc.

I told Angee of my positive impressions of the book and three days later found myself inquiring of her some knowledge of those soybean "meats" mentioned in the book that produce the same tastes as ham, hot dogs, chicken, steak, etc. "Now what the dickens made my tongue and brain ask such a dumb question?"

Angee responded by inviting me on a vegetarian picnic. I accepted only on the condition (I'm serious) that I be allowed to bring a couple bottles of wine because 'I'll have to be drunk to eat that stuff." Angee just chuckled and said something like "Don't knock it until you've tried it."

I'll never forget that picnic day. Angee showed up with her large picnic basket with a red table cloth covering it, looking every bit the part of Red Riding Hood. And I felt like the Big Bad Wolf, of course. She had taken careful measures to fix a variety of typical vegetarian offerings. I could not believe my taste buds! EVERYTHING was delicious and I got all of the positive taste sensations that I had received for years from conventional American and Foreign cuisines—yet 1) I had no grease or cholesterol; 2) I had no refined sugar; 3) I had no fat; 4) I had relatively few calories; 5) There were no dangerous food additives; and 6) I did not have that "bloated" feeling afterwards that I, and most obsessive-compulsive eaters, experience after most every "sitting." Quite frankly, I was dumb-founded—and decided that very day (conversion?) to become a vegetarian! Because, most imporant, I had received THE SAME EMOTIONAL SATISFACTION from the all-vegetarian meal—and that's the key for the foodaholic—because foodaholism IS an emotional problem. I've emphasiz-ed that throughout this book because I want you to MAKE NO MISTAKE ABOUT IT! Your problem is not just an organic one—no matter how hard you try to convince yourself or someone else tries to convince you.

Over the next few weeks and months, I learned quickly that there is just as much physical and emotional satisfaction in consuming a plate of raw broc-coli dipped in low calorie ranch dressing as there is in "inhaling" a plate of hot peanut butter cookies with two large glasses of milk; that "Wham" is just as good as ham; and that vegetable-cheese casseroles, properly prepared, are purely as pleasing to the palate as my Mother's classic swiss steak, gravy, mashed potatoes, homemade rolls, and ranch cake dinner. By the way, I still eat that meal every year on my birthday to show myself that I'm not "neurotic" and fanatic about this whole vegetarian bit. And I'm informing you of same so that you don't think me a hypocrite. But, by golly, I don't do it very often!

I want to also mention that I do eat chicken, turkey, and other meats of the bird and various foods of the sea such as shrimp, crab, oysters, etc.—but never fried! Therefore, I am not what would be defined as a pure vegetarian—but I'm close, and I truly love it! I literally feel better, both physically and psychologically, than I felt at 20, 25, 30, 35 and 40 years of age. Our basic diet in this country is terrible—and wasteful, and indulgent, and destructive. And yes, in my opinion, immoral and inhumane!

LET'S
TALK MORALITY, MOTHER!

I mentioned earlier that I never tasted an alcoholic drink until I was 30 years old. When I did finally begin to drink a few beers, my

Mother, a very strict moralist, became quite indignant and judgmental of my newly-found "sinful" vice. My protests fell on deaf ears as she quoted me biblical phrases ranging from "Do not drink strong drink" to "Do not destroy the temple which God gave you to house your soul."

This latter quote was particularly interesting to me since I was watching my own father quickly self-destructing HIS "temple" through extreme food abuse and my own mother was a major contributor to it. In addition, she herself was grossly overweight. Yet, when I would point out her and Dad's "sinful" behavior, she didn't wish to hear it. In fact, at least to me, she always either denied Dad's behavior as SINFUL, or rationalized that the Lord "understood" his problem. Yet, she never conceded that possibly He could "understand" my six beers per week (at that time) "problem."

My intent here is not to be critical of my mother. It is to point out that, in my opinion, gross obesity is a moral issue and that truly fat people should "judge not lest they be judged." It is my belief that destroying the body by the abuse of food is just as "sinful" as any other behavior—with the exception of "sins" which destroy others rather than self. Therefore, if you are a fat moralist—that is, a grossly overweight sermonist, I don't want to hear it from you. Clean up your own act first!

Let me tell you of one more major example of mysterious thinking before we move on—though I could recount hundreds of examples in my life. By this time, with my near-vegetarianism and daily exercise program, the pounds were melting quickly and my life was changing so quickly (to be discussed later in relationship to you). From 292 to 280 to 270 to 265, etc., though remember that I rarely weighed myself, as should you.

But also keep in mind that I am a middle-age man and gravity always takes its toll through the years. Therefore, my neck, upper arms, breasts, belly, hips, and butt were quite saggy—and my new self-concept found that altogether unacceptable. Aging is one thing, but benign neglect is a whole different ballgame.

I had always—even while a high school and college athlete—found weight lifting, nautilus, etc. very objectionable. I avoided it like the proverbial plague. So that was one area I absolutely would not get into, I thought, regardless of what my "mysterious thinking" tried to do to me, right? Wrong! Here's how THAT happened.

On our campus at Shawnee State College, we have a man named Harry Weinbrecht who serves as Athletic Director and Director of Health, Physical Education, and Recreation. I have known Harry for many years and watched him become an "expert" in Kinesiology (study of muscles, physiologically and anatomically) and the methods of building and maintaining the muscular structure of the body. Harry, himself, is an excellent physical "specimen" who constantly practices what he preaches and teaches. Frankly, he is probably the best built, fittest man over 50 years old that I've ever met.

So one day in the midst of my "mysterious thinking" era, I was in the gymnasium while Harry was working out with a set of free weights. Suddenly, I am "mysteriously" telling Harry of my sagging body parts and asking him if there is a program he could recommend (well, slap my face!) that might firm up said body parts. Harry answered "certainly!" and proceeded to show me a strenuous program combining free weights, universal machines, and nautilus apparatus. His very demonstration of the work-out tired me so much that I just went home and went to bed. NO WAY was I going THAT far. I've always felt that those types of work-outs represented too much narcissim (self-worship) and vanity, anyway. Leave that stuff to the macho men!

Yep, you guessed it, one week and seven tri-lateral programming sessions later I was in the gym huffing and puffing with Harry's "crazy" work-outs—and have been doing so ever since. You would not believe the results. My arms are big and firm; my butt is; my belly is "almost" hard and flat; and my "boobes" don't sag too much given 46 years of Mr. Newton's discovery. In other words, I ain't to bad—for an old codger.

Those are just three of my episodes of "mysterious thinking." There are hundreds of others and they've turned my life from "quiet desperation" to "fun and challenging." All this (and more yet to come in this book) is yours for the asking—or for the tri-lateral programming. If life is to be anywhere near meaningful, it must be an on-going process of growth and development. Tri-lateral program will make your life just that.

DON'T THINK VANITY

There is a thin line between self-pride and vanity. But it is an easily discernible line and an important one for you to recognize and avoid crossing. Just as there is a fine line between quiet confidence and obnoxious cockiness—you know what I mean. It is one thing to know that you look as nice as you can look and that you are taking pride in your appearance. It is another to have a semi-delusion of grandeur in which you begin flaunting and seeing yourself as "God's gift to _____!" It is one thing to be realistic and humble within yourself and another to be unrealistic and ostentatious (overt showiness).

The latter in all the above examples simply proves that you are still highly insecure within yourself and your progress—therefore your progress is insignificant and non-productive. You would ALMOST be better off to remain obese than to become vain with your slenderness. Vanity and narcissim show that you either haven't conquered your obsessive-compulsive actions or at least haven't learned to channel them properly for your own success.

Just keep in mind a statement I coined a decade ago: "Your life (and mine) is at the same time highly significant and highly insignificant." It is significant because you count; because you are a magnificent creation of the universe over millions of years; because you are a highly intelligent being that can consciously make your own decisions and think in the abstract; because you are you and only go around one time before your ashes go back to the ashes—your dust back to the dust. Go get 'em, important person! Don't fear to try anything you wish—to dream your dreams and work hard to make them come true. This is the essence of life! Forget 95% of society's guilt trips.

But don't forget—EVER—that you are highly insignificant, also. Life is like a "breeze passing over a field of wheat" and you are but a grain of sand on the cosmic beach. Few people care whether you live or die and even fewer will have their lifestyle altered ONE BIT if you die right now. That's the way it is and that's the way it has to be. When I see any person—famous or infamous—who sees himself larger than life, with an exaggerated perception of his importance within his immediate environment, I grow sympathetic and think "You poor miserable creature. Who the hell do you think you are? If you passed away right now, you have me confused with someone who'd really give a damn." I've met many of them, haven't you? Don't fall into the vanity trap! Your job, your community, and even your family will hardly miss a beat if you pass away right now. So how can you or anyone, think that you (they) are indispensible?

OTHER USES
OF TRI-LATERAL PROGRAMMING

I have many students and clients ask if these 20 minute creative imagery sessions can be utilized for other change besides weight loss-weight control—and if so, what? The answer is obviously "absolutely." And the sky is the limit as to whatever mental and emotional alteration you desire. Within physical limitations, you can program yourself to any goal. For example, no matter how hard you fantasize, if you are 5'4'' you won't become the pivot man for the Lakers. No matter how much tri-lateral programming I do, I won't look like Tom Selleck or Burt Reynolds. HOWEVER, with said tri-lateral work, you WILL become the best basketball player you can possibly become and I WILL become the best looking man I can possibly become. That's all that really matters.

Let me present some quick examples of what you CAN do with tri-lateral programming of your own computer:

A) WANT TO BE WEALTHY?

That's an easy one. Why? Because making money is one of the easiest things to do in a basically free, capitalistic economy. I'll show you how later—but for the time being, trust me. It's as easy as falling off a log.

We're back to internalized self-concept again. You show me a person who isn't well-to-do, and I'll show you a person who doesn't truly wish to be. He simply pays lip-service to it just like the athletes and rationalizing foodaholics already discussed—meanwhile hoping he wins the state lottery or that a rich relative dies and dumps a bundle in his lap. If he REALLY had an image of himself as wealthy he'd either be wealthy by now or be well on his way.

Have you ever heard of the old saying, "Poor people have poor ways." It's true and it represents the ultimate self-concept statement. They are poor because they have an internalized image of being poor and therefore continually, diligently, and relentlessly work to remain poor. If you are lower middle income; or middle income; or whatever income—then that's how you see yourself. Do you really want to change? It'll cost you 20 minutes per day and some highly creative, organized imagery—plus one more technique coming in the next session—and you'll be on your way. You just cannot believe how easy making money is if you TRULY desire to and learn the simple techniques.

You won't believe how the "mysterious thinking" will grab you on this one. There are thousands of possibilities and the money-making game is fascinating if you're REALLY into it. Does it take much intelligence? Nah! Many of our wealthiest people are below the norms on any given intelligence measure. There is a great deal of research over the years to support this simple fact.

After a given period of time and given number of sessions, all types of mysterious thinking will occur. For example, whereas before you might have stopped at a Dairy Queen for an ice cream cone, now you'll "mysteriously" find yourself wondering if that Dairy Queen is for sale; noting its excellent location; inquiring if it might be for sale if the price is right; researching financing methods, etc. And if its purchase seems reasonably feasible to you, you'll soon buy it. "Just what the hell will I buy it with?" you ask? Don't worry, "mysterious" will find a way. You'll see!

Whereas before you had passed a home with a "For Sale" sign and thought nothing of it, you might now pass that same home and discover yourself noting its location and the potential for dividing it into apartments and renting it. The sub-dividing of land—and buildings—have been two of our major creators of great wealth in this country. Prime example: Picture the square footage of a small hotel room in a thriving city. That room rents for, let's say $62.00 per night. That adds up to $1,860.00 per month rent for that small space. Lawsy me, lawsy me! You can rent an apartment bigger than that for $250.00 monthly. But, at the same time, picture a house that would rent for $300.00 a month and break even on mortage payments. Alter it into four decent apartments; rent them for $250.00 monthly—$1,000.00 total—and you profit $500.00-$700.00 per month. See how easy it is? Many below average intelligent men and women have made big money at this sub-division game for decades. Buying farms and sub-dividing them into lots or mini-farms is just like mining gold. If you REALLY wish to make money, it is so simple. I'll give you more examples later.

But the major point here is that almost all wealthy people have one major psychological characteristic in common: A deep intensive need to be wealthy—in other words, they think about it (mental imagery) almost continually. They love to make money, count money, horde money, and the power/prestige money brings. Get the self-concept message? Their internalized self-image is "Big-Time" so their entire being relentlessly works toward becoming "Big-Time." That's why failures and bankruptcies don't phase them in the least.

B) "I'M SHY
AND WANT TO BE MORE ASSERTIVE"

O.K., then your tri-lateral programming should daily be oriented to picturing yourself in situations in which you once "stayed back" but now are stepping forward. Combined with the technique to be discussed next, you will soon find yourself performing some strange (mysterious) actions. For example, let's say that you even have difficulty making eye contact and speaking to people while in a public setting (many people do). How pleasantly surprised you'll be (you may have to slap yourself in the face) when you "mysteriously" find yourself starting to do so. And keep up your tri-lateral programming—plus the next recommendation—and you'll begin to quickly blossom like a beautiful flower. Stepping up to front and center will get in your blood and you'll be hooked on it. Heck, you'll be asserting yourself all over the place.

C) "MY AGGRESSION WORKS AGAINST ME"

This is a very common problem which, unfortunately, most people don't even know they suffer. Because overt aggression is so threatening to those around us, high-aggression persons who display same are rarely successful. Their peers work against them being successful! And since they treat others aggressively, they usually treat themselves aggressively also—and therefore self-destruct. If I had more time, I could write an entire chapter on this "aggression syndrome," but for the present, believe me that high-aggresion persons are usually their own worst enemy.

But for those fortunate few who do perceive their excessive aggression (the great significance of Socrates' "Know Thyself" insight) and TRULY wish to change, tri-lateral programming, plus what comes next, is invaluable. First, remember that aggression to a psychologist is defined as "overcoming opposition forcefully." The term is often misused by laymen to describe people who have high achievement needs—"He is aggressive in his ambition."

So, if you have a "chip on your shoulder" too often; realize same; and truly wish to change; the techniques contained in this book will work for you. Simply picture yourself being non-aggressive (end result) in situations in which you have habitually been aggressive and take the "medication" to be recommended next, and you'll soon be on your way toward becoming SUPER COOL in most every setting. Your aggression toward others will either decrease significantly or you will at least learn to "channel" your aggression to work FOR rather than against you. I know. I've been down that road before, too. I used to get my back in the air and would come out swinging everytime I was backed into any psychological/emotional corner. How dumb I was—and how much time and potential I wasted.

CONCLUDING STATEMENT

If you do your tri-lateral programming EVERY DAY for 20 minutes, your "mysterious thinking" will become so frequent that it will astound you. I have not found ONE EXCEPTION in those who participate faithfully. Your life will quickly begin to take on depth and dimensions that you had never previously thought possible. The remainder of this book (not counting the next super chapter) will help you to handle all the positive changes that you'll experience.

CHAPTER ELEVEN

Now For Your Diet Pills!

At this point in my program, I usually shock my clients—and probably you—by informing them that our endeavors will not be successful unless they agree to take "diet pills" each day, EVERY DAY for a long time to come. Just as tri-lateral programming has changed the entire direction of my life, so has my pill taking. I must inform you that I am "hooked" on pills—yes, very much pill dependent—and I sincerely believe that you CAN-NOT be successful in my program without them. Therefore, assignment #10, and the last of my FIRM assignments, is that you MUST take pills SIX times per day for a long period of time—again, as though your life depends on them, because it does! Laugh if you must, though I cautioned you not to. Call it "silly" if you desire—though you agreed not to. Your life-long change is based upon tri-lateral programming and "pill-taking." Are you up to it? It's quite easy and fun, but there are specific instructions you need to follow. After you have reached your target weight, you will be able to stop taking pills. But you'll probably discover you'll wish to take alternate pills to reach alternate goals. Before I give you your "pills," let's first review your SPECIFIC directions for their intake:

1) Secure an empty pillbox or small vitamin bottle. I highly recommend the vitamin bottle because of the social stigma of taking REAL drugs and that, due to your daily life pattern, it is inevitable that eventually people may discover you taking your "pills."

2) Get a neatly-cut slip of paper and print your "pills" on that sheet of paper.

3) Literally go through the physical motions of taking a pill (water and all—including the hand motion of sticking the "pill" in your mouth. This becomes even more effective as time passes due to the tremendous psychological symbolism involved). Admittedly, the six glasses of water per day serve a purpose, also—especially in the beginning—but they serve no long-range purpose and are not meant to subtlety get you on a water diet.

4) Take these "pills" as religiously as though a doctor has prescribed them for your very survival—such as insulin, heart pills or blood pressure pills. When I relate to you the results these pills have produced in me (and many others), you'll either be astounded or completely convinced finally that I'm BONKERS. However, if you take these SIX pills SIX times daily—and do your tri-lateral programming daily—a new, wonderful life is in your near future. If you conveniently forget to take them, then you are again searching for excuses to lose.

THE SIX "DIET PILLS"

They are so simple, yet it took me quite a while to perfect them and place them in proper order to derive maximum effects. The wording of them is carefully designed for maximum effect and the emotional nature of your wording is crucial. I'll explain this soon.

PILL #1

To be taken every morning BEFORE breakfast. Remember to drink water, while symbolically placing this "pill" in your mouth. Then read from your pillbox sheet this "pill:" "I AM TRULY ENJOYING BEING SLENDER." Do so with great emotion—I'll show you why in the next section. Soon you'll memorize all six of your mental diet pills but continue ALWAYS to take your pill container out and literally go through the action of taking a pill. I've been doing it for FOUR YEARS and I'll relate some of my great experiences with them later.

Obviously, Pill #1 is worded in the present tense purposely. I began taking this "pill" when weighing 292 lbs.—and hardly enjoying being slender—but these pills are just another phase of your programming. You must begin to see yourself as slender before your cerebral cortex and limbic system will lead you DILIGENTLY and doggedly in that direction. And the word "enjoying" is a very emotional word. Put special emphasis upon it to yourself, even if you have to be dramatic and theatrical about it.

PILL #2

Pill #2 is a follow-up of pill #1 and should be taken religiously at mid-morning—approximately 10:00 A.M. Again, take with water and symbolically "pretend" you're taking a pill while repeating, "IT'S REALLY ENJOYABLE TO BE SLIM AND TRIM." Also, again talk to yourself with deep emotion—even theatrically. Place emphasis this time on "really," "enjoyable," "be" (present tense), and "slim and trim."

Note that this "pill" not only re-inforces #1 but also adds the "trim" factor. This assures that you'll soon "mysteriously" also seek body definition through exercise and the fitness regimen already discussed. Body definition will be discussed soon and it will become just as important to you as the actual weight-loss. After a few weeks (usually six), Pill #2 will carry you quite handily from 10:00 A.M. to lunch with no "hankering" to work toward obesity—only slenderness.

PILL #3

To be taken EVERY DAY BEFORE lunch is this wonderful diet pill: "IT'S NICE TO HAVE PRIDE IN MYSELF AND MY PERSONAL APPEARANCE." This is my second most favorite pill and the cumulative effect of this instrument of "internalization" has had a great influence upon my life. After six weeks of pill #3—plus, of course, my 20 minute tri-lateral programming—I found it almost impossible to over-eat ("pig-out"), even when I tried to do so. I mean that!

It first began by "mysteriously" affecting my lunch habits. I slowly but surely progressed from a two hamburger, french fries, milkshake lunch to a one hamburger, glass of milk, salad lunch—then to a salad and fruit juice lunch—without even realizing the metamorphosis (change). It was amazing and it was wonderful. I began feeling better not only physically—but emotionally. The "bloated" and sluggish feelings disappeared almost immediately and my energy level increased significantly. You're going to fall in love with Mister Mystery!

This pill soon led me not only to better eating and exercise habits—but to a whole new world of SEARCHING DILIGENTLY for better ways to improve my personal grooming and dress procedures. I will discuss this more in the last section of the book, but I must tell you now that I discovered an entire new, challenging world in clothes and how to wear them properly—and in grooming techniques. I had always been clean previously, and reasonably well-dressed and groomed. But I soon realized (with the solicited help of Angee Whitt) that I had only touched the surface. I discovered that "clothes truly do make the person" in so many different ways—the way people see you, treat you, relate to you—AND EVEN WORK FOR YOU AND YOUR SUCCESS. Oh, if I had only known how true this is 25 years ago. It would have been invaluable to me—just as my discussion of it later COULD WELL PROVE INVALUABLE TO YOU!

It has nothing to do with vanity or "dressing to the teeth" all the time. It has to do with pride; looking as well as one can look; and success-type thinking and behavior. I am deeply indebted to the instruction of Angela Yvonne Whitt in these areas. She is flat-out an expert in both male and female appearances. And don't you as a reader think for a moment that grooming and dress isn't highly significant—or that you can't ALWAYS find ways to look better—no matter how good you presently look!

We'll go into detail later. But, in the meantime, let me relate another classic example of "mysterious thinking" that happened to me after taking pill #3 for 12 weeks. I was in a department store in which a rather effeminate looking man was making a presentation on male colognes and perfumes. He was surrounded by all women. Three months previous, I would have gone by this guy like a freight train passing a tramp. But I mysteriously paused. Then I heard him make a statement that it was important for men or women to select scents that matched their body chemistries. Heck, I thought, anyone knows you simply wear Mennen Skin Bracer or whatever you get for Christmas. What's this guy mean when he says "experiment and probe until you find a scent compatible with your body oils, hormones, glands, etc.?" Was this namby-pamby serious?

But I listened—and I learned. He was right, and now I know it. One can find scents that combine with his personal aromas and that are beneficial to him. And the test is the number of people who tell you that you smell nice. Because one's smell is so personal that seldom—if ever—will someone tell someone else that they smell nice if they don't. And when you do smell well, MANY people will tell you. That same day I purchased the book HOW TO DRESS FOR SUCCESS (Me? Well, slap my face!) and attended a male style show in that same department store. Three months previous I would have thought all these sissyish. But there I was—and I'm a better man because of it. More to come later! But don't tell me—or most of my clients—that these pills don't work. They will grab the very fabric of your being—if you take them faithfully EVERY DAY!

PILL #4

"I THINK I'LL SEARCH FOR EVEN MORE AND NEWER WAYS TO MAKE MYSELF ATTRACTIVE AND SUCCESSFUL." This is a great pill and one which will assure you an ever dynamic and fresh future—the remainder of your life. I have seen the constant partaking of this pill actually work "miracles" and near-miracles in my own life and the lives of my clients. Take it in mid-afternoon, approximately 3:30 p.m.

Once you have internalized this "pill" (statement), your unconscious mechanism embodied in your cerebral cortex and limbic system will move you toward "mysterious" goals that will both dumbfound and confound you—in a highly positive manner. Let me give you some real-life examples. All of the following are true either of me or someone with whom I've worked. Naturally, the names have been changed simply to protect confidentialities. I have letters on file from these people which attest to their authenticity. The entire program, obviously, precipitated these changes—but each person has placed special emphasis on pill #4. I could relate lengthy and detailed stories of each person but will purposely be brief and "outline-ish."

A) TIM CELLERS

Tim was one of the first people to participate in my program—almost eight years ago. He was 5'9", 285 lbs., and very poorly groomed. His self-concept and ego strength were almost nil. He usually didn't even smell very well; he had moved from one menial task job to another; he was a 30-year-old bachelor and largely anti-female; and he was held in little regard in the community except for sympathy and the fact that he was described by most of the citizenry as a "pretty nice boy." Quite frankly, he closely fit the description of the poor self-concept, cowering dog described in my Lassie parable.

I watched this 30-year-old urchin "boy" emerge into one of the leading "men" in that community. More important, he watched it—and singled out the program contained in this book generally and pill #4 specifically as the major factors in his caterpillar-to-butterfly metamorphosis.

Today, Tim Cellers is a slender, well-built (defined), 180 lb. man; married with two children; vice-president of personnel of a leading company; an officer in two leading civic service clubs; challenged and happy in his lifestyle; and still growing.

Tim is admittedly one of the more dramatic turn-arounds of my tri-lateral programming and pill-taking program—plus what is to come in the next section—but there are many, many others. Incidentally, each year Tim writes me a letter of gratitude and sends me gracious Christmas gifts—too gracious! I return them—against his objections, as he states: "I would pay anything I had for what your program of self-concept did for me. I only wish I'd met you when I was 20 instead of 30. But 30 was good enough and 60 wouldn't even be too late." I still count this fine young man as one of my closest friends.

B) JOE EVANS

Joe is another of my favorites because his life also changed so drastically. Joe was 6'6" and well over 300 lbs. when he came to see me. He was a high school teacher-coach and was having great difficulty fulfilling his duties due both to his physical bulk and emotional guilt stemming from his gross overweightness. He had withdrawn from any social life or relationships with the opposite sex—opting to escape into the fantasy world of books. He walked with an exaggerated stoop and wore only XXX large velour shirts and "tent-like" pants. He perspired profusely and no amount of deodorants or colognes could cover it. His job was in jeopardy and his life miserable and quietly desperate when he sought me out.

He followed my program faithfully and also told me six months later that pill #4—in his opinion—was the highlight of the program and initiated more "mysterious" actions within him than any other pill. (I must tell you now that pill #4 is nevertheless not my favorite. I'll discuss it soon.)

I saw Joe Evans completely change his life—literally to a 360 degree turnabout. Within the next four years, Joe lost 145 lbs.; changed his walk to erect; attained a Masters degree—then a Ph.D. in Psychology; dated and fell in love with a wonderful woman; etc. He presently is a well-groomed, noted college professor in a major university in this country; has vast outside business interests; two beautiful children; and his life is exciting and significant.

Joe and I are close friends. I have become close to almost every client with whom I have worked personally. And, as I mentioned previously, the reason I'm writing this book in such a personal style is to attempt to be as intimate with you as is possible through a book—which obviously is limited. Joe and Tim did nothing that you also cannot do.

C) BRENDA JONES

Brenda is a classic example of something I do which I have not told you about. Periodically, when the occasion seems proper, and when I encounter a foodaholic that I'm certain would be highly attractive if he/she were slender and well-defined, I approach that person and tell them so. I then encourage him/her to participate in my program. While this may seem like crass salesmanship on my part, it really isn't. I don't really need the money because, as stated previously, I lead a very simple life-style. Admittedly, like most humans, I do enjoy the acceptance and gratitude of people once they have confronted and conquered foodaholism through my program—and I do like the prestige and status of being recogized as an authority in the area of weight loss-weight control. But I can tell you with all genuineness that my major satisfaction is watching that individual's glee as they become very beautiful right in front of their own eyes. Such is the case with Brenda Jones.

Brenda was a student of mine. She was 5'5'', 220 lb. blonde butterball. She had been a foodaholic since she was a child. But I noticed that all her features, most of which were covered by layer upon layer of fat, were flat-out fantastic. She had beautiful hair and eyes; high cheekbones and great facial bone structure; super complexion; full breasts; and a butt that you could set a Coke on and not spill a drop. The only problem was she needed to weigh 120 instead of 220. By the way, she was only 19 years old.

I felt I knew her well enough to tell her everything I just wrote above. In addition, I urged her to participate in my program so that she wouldn't spend her prime years of life as I had—grossly overweight—and then regretting it greatly in later years.

She readily agreed to work with me and over the next four months paid me $575.00. (In case you wish to know, I charge $25.00 per hour of counseling. I like to remind people that few plumbers will work a full hour in your home for less and most mechanical work on cars will cost $26.00 or more per hour simply for labor. I further remind them that the work I do, if effective, is much more significant to their lives than plumbing or cars. If not effective, I return their money.)

I have a letter on file from Brenda stating: "Looking back now, I would have paid you $20,000 for what you taught me. The changes that took place allowed me to recover the $575.00 within two months—$575.00 that I earned which I never would have with my previous outlook. I could never re-pay you enough."

Well, you should see her now. She lives in Orlando, Florida and is now 22—5'5", 120 lbs.—and an absolute "knock-out" in all her clothes, including bikini. As you'll see soon, I teach more than just how to conquer foodaholism and one thing I teach is how one can use his/her "sexualness" (not sex) to gain most any goal he/she desires. Brenda Jones has done just that. She loves her new life; is well on her way to becoming a millionaire through business entrepreneurship; and tells me she still takes pill #4 every day. Don't tell Brenda that the "pills" seem childish and/or silly. She knows what results their internalization brings and the direction in which they lead you.

D) JODY SMITH

Jody's case is similar to Brenda's but contains some different facets worth mentioning. She also had all very beautiful features, and I also approached her first. But whereas Brenda had been shy and retiring, Jody was the classic "jolly fat girl"—using her joviality as a defense mechanism to cover her hurt and shame, as 95% of jolly fat people are doing. In any event, Jody was an outgoing, gregarious person with a wonderful personality and I saw in her the potential to truly "conquer the world" if she so desired—which she does, as it turns out.

When I first knew her, she was 23 years old, 5'7", 235 lbs. She had worked a few jobs (unhappily), had no money, and had returned to school on a government grant. She also had no direction and did not even know what field she wished to enter. She drove an old junker car which broke down as often as it ran. However, that old car did give me great insights into her basic make-up, because she could always quite readily repair her car on her own and get it running.

To prove what I said earlier about my low priorities on money, I let her into my program free of charge (by the way, I only work with eight people per period—five months—all on a one-to-one basis. So I have time for only eight. My teaching, writing, lecturing, and seminar-conducting consume the remainder of my time. I have a long waiting list. Quite frankly, my own tri-lateral programming and pills have led me into writing so prolifically that I will probably not return to counseling.

Jody has been magnificent! First, she used tri-lateral programming and the "pills" to reach a svelte 130 lbs. During this time, she used the pills and the next section of the book to decide upon a nursing career; became a head nurse in a hospital unit; arranged financing for her own nursing home, etc. She is presently proceeding "full speed ahead" to a chain of nursing homes and you should watch her "smoke." She's brilliant! It was all there—and everything fell in place as she went through my program. I love watching her!

E) GIAVONNA

Giavonna is very possibly my prize pupil. She approached me now almost four years ago. I could discuss her the remainder of this book but will be as brief as possible. Don't ever tell her that the various Walkian Formulas presented in this book do not work. You'd be in big trouble.

She was very plump but not grossly overweight (remember 30 lbs. or more than what one should weigh) and not really a foodaholic (which re-inforces my contention that this book is good for ANYONE to read). She had the potential to be one of the most beautiful women I've ever seen. I mean that—literally a Hollywood-type. I often referred to her as my Natalie Wood—woman.

She said she wished to enter my program and I told her that I didn't really think she was a foodaholic. She stated that she was but was fortunate to burn up a lot of it. She stated further that she had heard about the second part of my program (soon to come) anyway, and thought it would help her. I agreed, but told her I couldn't start her until the next session—three months hence.

I saw her a few times on a casual basis during that three months waiting period and learned much about her. She carried approximately 135 lbs. on a 5'5" model's frame that would make her a "convertible rider" at 110. Her potential for stunning beauty was obvious, and most of us are just not blessed in such a manner.

She was living with an older divorced man who, while good-looking and nice enough, was stifling her and "killing her with his song." He lived in a mobile home and had the "keep them barefoot and pregnant" philosophy. He was also a highly dominating, jealous, possessive man who was controlling most all of her actions. Giavonna was a tender and naive person with little self-concept and was readily submitting to the tactics of this man. For all intents and purposes, she was a Geisha Girl and "dirty underwear washer" for him. He loved it, of course, but it soon became evident that she wanted far more out of her life, had all the tools to do so, but really didn't know how to go about it. She was miserable, knew she was miserable, and felt as though she was in an unsolveable maze and "leg-hold" trap.

She went through my five month program. I in no way tried to influence her except in my areas of expertise—conquering foodaholism and wholesome self-concept and how both lead to success. I don't attempt to influence any other decisions of any of my clients. It's their life, they lead it! In that respect, I would be considered very non-directive or client-centered in my counseling approaches.

I knew that she was a classic example of a woman who had accomplished little, experienced little, traveled little, and had no idea of her potentials to accomplish greatly, experience much, and travel widely—but I said nothing, on purpose. I wanted to see just how effective my principles would be with this particular young woman—then 18 years old. Well, I've never had anyone quite like her. She even sold me more on my own program than I had been sold previously. It would take a small booklet to detail all that has happened to her in the past four years so I'll simply summarize:

1) She was known as cute or "cutesy." She is now one of the more beautiful women in Ohio and the midwest. She is literally a "head-turner" every where she goes. Both men and women stop to admire her beauty. This was not so previously.

2) She then dressed nice enough. Now she is probably the best dressed woman in this area of Ohio—and spends minor amounts on clothes (I'll discuss this technique later). She always looks like "a million bucks," even in jeans and sweatshirt.

3) Like most young women, she only dreamed of being a model. Now she is one—and gets more requests than she can fill. I can name you 20 agencies east of the Mississippi who write or call her every week.

4) She had no career plans. Now she already has four careers in action: Nursing, modeling, seminar work, and business entrepreneurship. Her life and career are so challenging that she needs a private secretary just to keep her itinerary organized.

5) She had hardly traveled outside her home area. Now she has traveled all over the U. S. and will soon be going to both Europe and South America.

6) She soon decided to escape her mobile home "jail" and "warden" and is now engaged to a successful doctor—a man of quality and depth, a gentleman (gentle man) in every sense. He encourages and develops her growth rather than inhibiting it. How fortunate a woman (or man) is to have such a spouse. Believe me, many don't! Dominating, stifling husbands were always the major complaint I got in marriage counseling.

7) Then she mainly went bowling with her "man." Now she attends movies, plays, concerts, and reads. She now has depth as a woman, is enlightened educationally, and is a challenging conversationalist. Then she was highly intelligent, but shallow and uninformed.

I recently had lunch with her and she said (quote) "I owe it all to you and what I learned from you. I would have lived my entire life and would never have known my potentials and strengths or fulfilled my dreams. Now everyday I search for new ways to be attractive, successful, and use my mind (pill #4). God must surely have sent you to me.''

Well, I don't have delusions of grandeur and believe that God sent me to mold peoples' lives. But I do know that I have hundreds of letters saying similar things to me—and do believe that God gave me the insights I have so that I can help solve the greatest problem in the U. S. today—LACK OF SELF-CONCEPT DUE TO OBSESSIVE-COMPULSIVE EATING!

"TIME OUT"
FOR TIME EFFICIENCY!

On the previous page, I mentioned in #4 that Giavonna's life was so challenging and busy that she needed a private secretary to plan her itinerary. Most of you have heard the old axiom, "If you want a good job done, ask a busy person to do it." I am convinced that this is true, almost without exception, and that it is true, once again, simply due to the five principles of self-concept psychology that I presented earlier.

However, I want to relate a story (parable) to you now that has greatly changed my entire life-style. It also had a tremendous effect on Giavonna's. Before I told it to her, I forewarned her, AS I AM YOU, that it was a crude, bawdy old story told to me by my grandfather, but that it contains one of the deepest universal psychological truths known to man. I'll wager many of my male readers have heard this story, but I'll also bet they haven't "digested" the great significance of it.

An old bull and a young "stud" bull were standing on a high hill admiring all the beautiful, sensuous cows grazing down in the valley. Both were very erotically stimulated by the mass of pulchritude that was gathered in that grassy vale. (Whew, am I working to clean up this story!)

Suddenly, the young bull turned to the old bull and said in a macho, cocky, brash, confident, excited, emphatic voice, "Let's RUN Down there and "have our way" with one of those little "honeys."

The older, veteran bull remained silent for a few moments, slowly reached down and got himself a large clump of grass, slowly chewed on his cud for a while, nonchalantly turned his head toward "stud man," and softly drawled, "Son, let's WALK down and have our way with them all!"

Now, I warned you that it was crude and lewd. But what a message it contains for compulsive, impulsive, "neurotic," "spin your wheels" persons like many of you reading this book are. Slow down and accomplish more. Cool it and achieve more. Organize and conserve and you'll move ahead much more quickly.

PILL #5

EVERY DAY I AM BECOMING A BETTER HUMAN BEING"

This is a simple "pill" (used by many self-concept writers) that I put in the pill box to further re-inforce pill #4. It should be taken immediately before dinner, again emphasizing the emotionality of each word.

While the intent of Pill #5 is quite evident, and you'll soon find yourself unconsciously and mysteriously working to become a better human being EVERY DAY, it has an interesting side effect. That is, I guarantee you that you'll soon find yourself learning to RELAX more as you habitually take this "pill." Almost all my clients agree that this pill soon produces a deep feeling of well-being within them—and Pill #6 will even do it more so. And, as discussed previously, relaxed foodaholics simply don't eat as much as up-tight ones do. In fact, relaxation is the natural opposite of obsessive, compulsive. Therefore, as you become more and more relaxed, you are by nature more and more "cured." Pill #6 will soon add even more relaxation to your life. I guarantee it.

Pill #5 is also beginning to put the finishing touches on your new self-concept. It is highly important that you see yourself growing into a better human being each day. For we either grow and develop each day, or we go backward—atrophy and die—a little each day. There is no such thing as standing still or status quo when it comes to human growth and development. I am still in the process of becoming better each day—and you should be also. Integrate, don't disintegrate! Build, don't destruct! Live, not die! Enough said!

LET'S BRIEFLY DISCUSS FASTING!

Since I'm on the subject of relaxation and stress management, I want to take a few moments to discuss food fasting with you. Actually, I should have done so in an earlier chapter but it is quite appropriate at this point.

First, let it be said that fasting is not a part of the program presented here because I want no problems with the medical profession and would not want to endanger your health, if fasting would be damaging to your particular body. So you most certainly would want to check with your family physician before you follow this personal recommendation:

I have found that four or five fasts per year lasting about five days each are extremely purifying, relaxing, and stress-reducing for me. Interestingly, they have contributed little or nothing to my weight loss over a long period of time and I do NOT recommend fasting as a weight-loss tool. I simply believe in very limited fasts as psychological, emotional instruments. Though I cannot explain why, fasting provides me with a "rush" or "high" far superior to any artificially-induced one that I've ever experienced. Furthermore, on day #2, #3, #4, and #5, I increasingly take on more and more energy and truly take on a cleansed, purified feeling that is fantastic. After five days, at least for me, all these "benefits" begin to wane and disappear quickly.

Again, I cannot legally or ethically recommend fasting to you, but for me it is a super experience—except for day #1. For what it's worth, I drink a great deal of water and take mega-vitamin dosages during my fasting.

PILL #6

"I AM A TRULY FINE PERSON SO I CAN JUST RELAX AND ENJOY MY LIFE"

This is my favorite "pill" and it has worked a personal miracle in my life. It is to be taken every night immediately before going to bed. Usually, I take it while IN bed, and you'll soon see why I do so. I have been taking this pill for four years. It began to produce beneficial results after just SIX WEEKS and has gotten better ever since. It has changed my daily living patterns even more than the other five—and they're darn effective.

If you happen to be a high-guilt person, and many foodaholics are (it's one of the major causal factors of foodaholism), then you'll find that this pill will "mysteriously" begin to reduce your guilt levels after prolonged usage. Quite frankly, I recommend heavy dosages of this pill and often take it five or six times daily. I'll discuss why soon.

Many people don't understand guilt—either its definitions or its origin. Keep in mind that I have written a book on guilt, **GUILT—GO TO HELL!** It is out of print now (it sold over 30,000 copies), but I am presently revising it and titling it **GUILT—BE GONE!** The previous title scared many ultra-religious people from reading it. You can order it by sending $12.95 to me and the book will be in the mail within a few months. To a psychologist, guilt is defined in the same manner as its origin: **FEAR OF PUNISHMENT BY SOMEONE WHO HAS THE POWER TO RENDER YOU HELPLESS IN SOME MANNER BECAUSE YOU DID NOT MEASURE UP TO SOME CERTAIN SET STANDARD.** Every guilt feeling you experience is some form of the above.

Many people carry heavy guilt and it's quite burdensome. I call guilt the **THREE-D** emotion—the most degrading, destructive and debilitating of all the human emotions. Further, guilt of some type or another is the origin of ALL the other negative human emotions, in my opinion. It's also true that most of our guilt feelings (95%) are completely unnecessary. Yet, guilt will eventually eat you alive and spit you out. Therefore, many people are self-destructing through guilt (and usually the accompanying emotions) completely unnecessarily.

But Pill #6, I guarantee, will slowly but surely reduce your feelings of guilt if taken religiously. It will at the same time increase relaxation and reduce stress and tension. My ground rule for feeling guilt is quite simple: Anytime I knowingly hurt another human being, I do feel guilty. Other than that, you might as well forget laying a guilt trip on me because you're just wasting your time. I will simply lay my favorite guilt CURE line on you. "Perhaps, just perhaps, you're confusing me with someone who really gives a rat's ass." But at times we do knowingly hurt others—and we do feel guilt. Pill #6 will even help those times—AND IT WILL EVENTUALLY ERASE ALL OF YOUR UNNECESSARY GUILT. A wonderful gift from me to you is Pill #6—and all you have to do is take it once every night, though four or five times per day is better. Take it anytime you feel anxiety or "up-tight." After steady dosages for six weeks, it will become better for you than a dumptruck load of librium and valium.

Secondly, many of you foodaholics out there suffer from much body and/or head tension—just as I do. Therefore, it is difficult for you to relax—and possibly even to sleep, especially if you suffer from the depression and anxiety which usually accompanies guilt and/or gross overweightness. Then you'll soon find Pill #6 to be the greatest thing since indoor plumbing, sliced bread, Pepsi, and peanut butter—or in a more serious vein—the greatest thing since sleeping pills, librium and valium or booze. Because you can soon throw them away as relaxation or sleep aids (crutches).

THE MIRACLES!

When I was 30 years old—16 years ago—I experienced a moderate anxiety reaction, commonly called in slang terms, a mild "nervous breakdown." It is a neurotic reaction which I detail in my previous book—a high-anxiety episode which is both frightening and mentally/physically painful. The causes of my anxiety reaction were both organic (physical) and functional (guilt, driveness, burn-out, etc.) and I won't go into them here. Suffice it to say that this experience endured and plagued me significantly for two/three years and even as it subsided, and I taught myself to deal with it (which I did—I had no outside help), there were still some "residue" effects.

One of those was a very bothersome brain wave syndrome which left me with persistent head tension, vagus nerve over-stimulation (chest and heart-beat) and over-all body tension. I courageously—yes, even bravely—lived with this high tension pain for 10 years, seldom getting any sleep at night beyond fitful dozing due to finally just becoming exhausted. I made insomniacs look like Micky Mouse and Little League! All this was depressing and I saw days and nights that I thought would never end.

As mentioned previously, four years age I began the entire program included in this book—including, of course, Pill #6. I am living proof of what this entire sequence can do for you as are many others with whom I've worked, but I especially want to relate to you what Pill #6 "hath wrought" in my life. After taking this pill nightly for two months, I began to notice that most (not all) nights I was falling asleep more readily and sleeping a little longer each time (in my case, up to a full hour—which I had seldom done in a decade). I became like a child with a new toy! Unless you are a chronic insomniac, you could never know what a blessing I had discovered. I knew right then that I would never abandon Pill #6.

So, I began taking the pill during the day, anytime I felt up-tight (tension) about any particular daily happenstance. I soon noticed that symbolically going to a water fountain and taking this "pill" would literally relax my body and mind—only a little, but I could actually, physically feel the muscle and emotional "easing" take place. The relief was immediate—albeit slight—and I was overjoyed.

But what happened over the next six months overwhelmed me, and still does today. Simply believe what I tell you is true. There is no reason for me to lie to you. After all, you've already bought my book, anyway (ha)!

Now, I can take pill #6 at night in bed and IMMEDIATELY, yes IMMEDIATELY, go to sleep nine out of ten nights. I have "learned" (internalized the pill) to react to this phrase in the same manner as a "good subject" does to his hypnotist, that is, the hypnotist can soon get a trusting subject to go into a deep relaxation, hypnotic trance even with a key phrase and/or snap of the finger. This is true and it's one of the reasons many of you think some of the show business hypnotists you see on TV are fakes.

Nine out of ten nights, I can take my pill "JERRY, YOU ARE A TRULY FINE PERSON, SO JUST RELAX AND ENJOY YOUR LIFE" and accomplish the same. That is, I literally fall asleep immediately! By the way, you should know that my ideal night is spent in four, two-hour deep sleep sessions. I do not even enjoy sleeping eight hours straight. It makes my night seem too quickly over for me. Furthermore, I can also take Pill #6 during any stress period during the day, and almost without exception, derive immediate, complete relaxation! That is the truth, the whole truth, and nothing but the truth. I hope Pill #6 works the same "miracle" in your life. Take it faithfully. If it does work a psychological change within you, please write or call me and let me know.

TAKE PILLS WITH EMOTION, DRAMA, AND EVEN THEATRICS

As emphasized throughout this book, obsessive-compulsive eating is mainly an emotional problem. Remember the earlier section dealing with the importance of learning to derive emotional satisfaction out of slower eating; gaining similar emotional appeasement by substituting low calorie foods; and dividing portions for the psychological effects of bigger portions? In other words, it is the Limbic System (the house of emotions), along with the R-complex (hindbrain, instincts) that cause foodaholism, not the cerebral cortex (thinking cells). The cerebral cortex knows darn well that you don't need to keep eating potato chips or cashews even when you're no longer hungry. "Common sense" (cerebral cortex, rational, logical thinking) tells you that. But your emotional needs for food overrule all that, don't they? Therefore, the manner in which you take your six pills is very, very important. I'm very serious! You must not simply "go through the motions" with these pills. You must take them EMOTIONALLY so that the emotional internalization we seek within the limbic system will occur. And since you are talking to yourself—just as in the tri-lateral programming—the sky is the limit. Be creative, imaginative, dramatic, yes and even theatrical! Remember, all of life is a stage . . .

For example, I've given you your six pills. But let me show you how I take those same pills. You can "borrow" my way, if you wish, or create your own way—a formula (statement) which is suitable just for you.

Pill #1: "I really am enjoying being slender."

My Way:	(With sincere feeling—even theatrical actions in the beginning) "Man, oh man, I am truly enjoying being a slender, well-built man. It's wonderful—and it makes my life so beautifully different."
Pill #2:	"It's really enjoyable to be slim and trim."
My Way:	(Once more, with feeling) "I just love being slender and having hard body tone. It's a grrrreat way to live and enjoy life!"
Pill #3:	"It's nice to have pride in myself and my appearance."
My Way:	(With much MENTAL voice inflection—or ACTUAL voice inflection if I'm alone): "It's soooo' nice to constantly take pride in myself and to be proud of how I appear to others. It changes EVERYTHING for me. I'm so thankful that I've learned to do it."
Pill #4:	"I think I'll search for even more ways to make myself attractive."
My Way:	"The remainder of my life, I will always search for new ways to dress; new ways to groom myself, and ANYTHING that appears to make me a better man. That is the essence of success-type behavior."
Pill #5:	"Every day I am becoming a better human being."
My Way:	"Every day, in every way, I grow and develop as a person. It's exciting because I know I pass this way only one time. (Isn't it ironic that the best TV commercial ever made is a beer ad?: "You only go around one time. So do it with gusto!")
Pill #6:	"I am a truly fine person, so I can just relax and enjoy my life."
My Way:	"I have always been a good man and tried to be fair and just with people—attempting to treat them well, knowing I've made mistakes. But I do the best I can! So just relax, Jerry, and enjoy your life. It's the only one you have!"

IF YOU HABITUALLY TAKE THESE SIX PILLS WITH EMOTION—AND DO YOUR 20 MINUTE DEEP RELAXATION TECHNIQUE (TRI-LATERAL PROGRAMMING) FOR SIX WEEKS—AND HAVE NOT SEEN A SIGNIFICANT CHANGE IN YOUR LIFE AND DAILY ACTIONS—THEN YOU'LL KNOW THIS PROGRAM WILL NOT BENEFIT YOU AND THAT YOU ARE ONE OF THE 10% "INCURABLES." BUT THE ODDS ARE NINE TO ONE IN YOUR FAVOR. SO GO TO IT!!!

SOME COMMENTS
REGARDING ANOREXIA NERVOSA

As you may know, there is a common school of thought that America's alleged "obsession" with slenderness and weight loss is the major casue of our seemingly increase in the incidence of "Anorexia Nervosa"—that is, an obsessive-compulsive need NOT to eat and/or to be SKINNY! I think this is true—TO AN EXTENT (but only to a very small extent, as you'll see) and I'd like to give you my thoughts on this malady (emotional disease).

First, my experience and reading convinces me that the major cause of anorexia has little to do with America's emphasis on slenderness in the mass media, the modeling field, etc. Since the problem is largely confined to teenage and young adult women, it seems obvious that this disease goes far deeper than "fad" or mass media. If not, then men—and women of different age groups—would also suffer it more often.

I believe that most true anorexics have deep psychoanalytical origins. It is my belief (and I do not have the space to detail all this) that the majority of teen-age female anorexics have had (and it probably still persists) either a highly dominating male figure (usually a father) in their lives or a female (usually a mother) who is highly masculine. This dominating, possessive "man" has served as a "bleacher father" or "stage door mother" type—highly controlling the physical and psychological environment of the girl—yet not providing, from the beginning, the emotional warmth, peace, quietness, gentleness, and intimacy that the child needs. Usually the parent did not consciously mean to create this "cold fish" atmosphere, but they did. Therefore, as the young woman enters puberty with a significant lack of ego strength and affection, anorexia becomes her vehicle of complete REGRESSION—that is, her unconscious obsessive need to return to girlhood, even babyhood, in order to seek that of which she is deprived.

There is much evidence of this—not the least of which is the fact that as she loses sizable amounts of weight, her breasts disappear and the menstrual cycle ceases. She literally returns to being a little girl. So it is my contention that most anorexia is an exaggerated, deprivation, regression need.

However, I do also believe that America's obsession with slenderness is a significant factor. Let me explain because it offers even more credence (credibility) to my program. Foodaholics are obsessive-compulsive personalities, which is defined as a neurosis. They have developed psychic fixations, even libido (sexual) fixations, with food. Therefore, possessing this pre-disposition for extremes, it is quite easy for them to switch their extreme need to eat to an extreme need NOT to eat. Their life is marked by a strong tendency to multiply "normal" by 100—the best "home-made" definition of neurosis I've ever seen (I created it 20 years ago in graduate school).

All this is just another reason I don't believe much in fad diets, celebrity diets, crash diets, Weight Watchers, Physician's Weight Loss, etc.—and why I partially titled this book: THE ONLY WAY! You must program yourself away from extremity—that is obsessive-compulsive, neurotic behavior patterns.

In conclusion, people criticize (usually obese people) America's obsession with slenderness. Assuming they're right, all one must do is look around to find that we've certainly had an obsession with becoming fat then, also. Given a choice between obsessions, I'll select slender. But we also know that anorexics and bulimics (recurrent eating binges with induced vomiting) usually have problems far beyond just obesity concerns. That is why I put so much emphasis upon wholesome self-concept in this book.

TRI-LATERAL
PROGRAMMING FOR CHILDREN?

Is the tri-lateral programming just discussed a viable, workable program for obese children? Absolutely! In fact, the earlier the program is started the better. Naturally, a child that is very young is not ready or able to practice the steps because he cannot comprehend the concepts and principles of tri-lateral programming. In addition, he may not possess the attention span for semi-auto hypnosis.

However, in my opinion, a child at right-around nine years old is quite ready to practice an organized self-concept program such as this. And there are many children who are mentally and emotionally mature enough to even begin at six and seven years old.

If you have an obsese child or one who is showing distinct signs of becoming quite obese, talk with him (using words of his vocabulary level) about the principles of self-concept. Actually, you will find it easier to get him/her started in pre-puberty than post-puberty—when most children will, by nature, resist any program put forth by parents (authority figures). After discussing the program and principles with him—and observing closely his reaction—let him talk and LISTEN to him when he does.

Then show him how to put tri-lateral programming into practice and even work with him on it. You can use these techniques to cement your relationship with your child and to become his friend and counselor in the process.

A warning: Don't try to pressure or force him into these practices, just encourage, help, and "model" for him. You don't want to take away from his self-concept when the major purpose of the program is to enhance it. Actually, due to their great powers of fantasy, children may even profit from tri-lateral programming BETTER than adults. Children are believing creatures, you see. That's why many parents have them BELIEVING that they're no good, dumb, inferior, etc. So you can use my program to have them BELIEVING they are worthy, competent, and able to solve any problem. Problem-solvers always run the world!

AND HOW
ABOUT THE PILLS FOR CHILDREN?

The six psychological pills just discussed are SUPER for children. Everything I just said above regarding tri-lateral programming also applies to the pills EXCEPT I honestly believe they can even be started younger (even age five) provided the wording is further simplified so that the statements have meaning for them.

Who knows better than you how difficult it is to feel good about yourself as an adult if you haven't liked yourself very much as a child? Encourage your child to take these pills when he's young. When he's older, he may think they are "dumb" or "stupid," just as many of you do. But you are wrong!

ARE YOU READY?

If you participate conscientiously in the program outlined thus far, your life is about to change DRASTICALLY—for the better! Can you handle it? Surprisingly, many people can't. Their needs to wallow in their own desperation and defecation are simply TOO strong. They fear large-scale success. This is particularly true in women and much research has been conducted to prove same.

You will see changes that will overwhelm you. I will spend the remainder of this book showing you how to benefit from these changes. At this point, let me say that YOU CAN NOW RECOMMEND THIS BOOK TO ANYONE—INCLUDING NON-FOODAHOLICS. THEY WILL GET THEIR COMPLETE MONEY'S WORTH, AS YOU WILL JUST FROM WHAT IS WRITTEN STARTING HERE! One need not be overweight to profit from this entire book, and they certainly don't need to be obese to profit and benefit from Part III coming up.

PART III

NOW YOU'RE READY FOR SUCCESS!

CHAPTER TWELVE

The "New" You

In the past decade, I have worked with hundreds of obese persons and observed thousands more. In addition, I've specialized in eating disorders to the point that I would be considered somewhat of an authority on the subject. Along with parent-child relationships and self-concept psychology (interestingly, both closely related to foodaholism), obsessive-compulsive eating has become a major thrust of my career. During that 10 years, I have found, almost without exception, that two things happen when one begins to lose weight on a stable, steady basis:

1) Most of the other problems and negative aspects of your life begin to decrease. You find that, for some reason (and we both now know what it is), that your other hardships usually just begin to "dry-up" and slowly disappear much like a mud puddle dissipating in bright sunlight.

I can think of many women who have come to me for counseling and in the first two sessions each outlines a variety of problems. Typically, they relate problems such as A) Lack of repsect from their husband; B) Conflict with their children; and C) Disgusting interference from their mother-in-law as to parenting and "wife-ing." Now, let's just say that this client is quite obese—which often they are. And she may or may not have listed overweightness as one of her problems above. But whether or not she does, one of the first things I recommend is that she begin the basic program just discussed in Section II.

You should see some of the looks I get and hear some of the comments, "Look, I came here with different problems and now you want me to lose weight," or "Oh, you just want every obese person to enter your program," etc. But I still attempt to coax them into a daily regimen of weight-loss and let's hypothesize that they do start my program. Let's further hypothesize that we don't even further discuss their other problems, which often I don't. Well, you guessed it, it almost never fails that a few months later that woman will be telling me something similar to, "You know, Dr. Walke, I just can't believe how much more respect and consideration I'm getting from my husband now," or "Dr. Walke, my home is just not a "war zone" as it once was and the kids and I are getting along so much better," or "By gosh, I've been wanting to get firm with my mother-in-law for years and let her know, as nicely as possible, that it's my home and I darn well manage it—and the other day I told her just that." Believe me, I have witnessed this womanly metamorphosis many times. It almost always occurs in my program.

2) As a man or woman participates in the weight-loss through self-concept program, they will, again almost without exception, discover themselves becoming VERY MUCH MORE SUCCESS-ORIENTED AND DEVELOPING HIGHER ACHIEVEMENT NEEDS. Quite frankly, this often becomes a problem that must be dealt with because A) They are actually scared of high level success due to their previous poor self-image; and B) They often times begin to grow and develop BEYOND their spouse, fiance or boyfriend/girlfriend and their growth, self-fulfillment needs, and desire to be more fully human is an overt threat to their partner. I always try to warn both the client and their spouse/friend that this will probably occur once I see that the person is going to be successful in my program.

So, get ready for success! But what is success? Let's define it. Obviously, the word means different things to different people. But I assure you that no matter how you define it, YOU'LL SOON BE SEEKING IT!!!

Let's be honest. MOST people define success in terms of money and material wealth. If you do also, why apologize for it? Our great country is built upon rugged individualism (the harder you work, the more creative and/or intelligent you are, the more you get ahead). Rugged individualism is human nature—no matter how vehemently socialists and communists deny it. Incidentally, they practice it! Our unique country (first in the history of man) is also built on Capitalism—a philosophy of free enterprise and competitiveness which has brought by far the greatest progress in the history of man on this earth—probably a legacy of 3-5 million years. Therefore, even though Jesus Christ, and the figureheads of most of the world's religious sects, preached constantly against it, and possibly rightfully so, MATERIAL WEALTH is still our leading barometer of success. Even MOST of our

"Christian" protestant evangelists prove this axiom—as does the Catholic Church—a fantastic power structure and accumulator of material money and goods (I know I MAY have just alienated many Catholics—but what I did was just tell the truth. Are you going to hold that against me? Actually, most protestant churches are, unconsciously, just as pre-occupied with materialism).

FURTHER TRUTH SEEKING

Most of us do not consider ourselves successful unless we have money/property/goods to openly and ostentatiously show to others—or ourselves. And that's all well and good as far as I'm concerned. However, there are also many of you who define success as PEACE OF MIND AND SELF-ACCEPTANCE. I am one of you and believe this to be the most worthy of definitions. Obviously, there are many highly wealthy people who are miserable characters—ranging from business executives to entertainers; from movie stars to "Jet-setters;" and from sports heros to entrepreneuers due-to-inheritance. Many of you have readily recognized this and have come to terms with "success" as consisting of simple satisfaction with being a good husband or wife; serving as a wholesome parent; performing your job competently; being the best you can be within your personality—set limits; and belonging to the grass-roots persons who make it through the day with little mental/emotional turmoil. You have your "place in the sun" equal to the silver-spoons and you have the insights to recognize that "money does not bring happiness."

But there is also a sizable group of you who view "success" as gaining respect, prestige, and even power in your community through quality leadership and service, even though it may not carry material wealth along with it. This is also worthy because the "common herd" has always needed leaders of integrity in order to insure their lives, liberties, and pursuits of happiness. You, too, can be proud of your definition of "success." Greater love hath no person than to sacrifice his life style to gain the God-given freedoms for his brother. Loyal and honest politicians are such a "gift" to us, and so rare a bird. We are fortunate, in my opinion, to have such a proven great one where I live in Vernal Riffe.

But the point here is that, as you conquer your foodaholism and gain new self-concept, you will "mysteriously" search for new success—new ways to reach your potentials and attain success as YOU define it. It is my job in the remainder of this book to attempt to show you the SPECIFIC principles of doing so. THERE ARE DEFINITE WAYS THAT SUCCESSFUL PEOPLE THINK AND SPECIFIC ACTIONS THAT SUCCESSFUL PEO-

PLE TAKE! And all of you are making a major mistake if you don't realize that—whether or not you're obese.

"SUCCESS"
AS DEFINED BY JERRY L. WALKE

Quite frankly, my definition of success emcompasses all the above. Naturally, I like peace of mind and satisfaction with my job and daily living—because without these all other "triumphs" are empty and meaningless. Ask Judy Garland, Elvis Presley, Marilyn Monroe, Freddy Printz, Howard Hughes, etc. How miserably tragic it would be to conquer the world—at least within your field of endeavor—and yet self-destruct within your own conflict and turmoil. But millions have throughout the history of mankind.

Also, I desire the respect of my peers and colleagues and the prestige within the community that goes with it. Note that I did not mention "power." I've never been too bent on dominating and controlling others and need very little power over others in my lifestyle. I'm often interpreted this way because of my high exhibition needs (ostentation and flamboyancy) but I've never been a very dominating person. That's why I'm not really a very effective or willing leader—and never have been. I've "held my own" in leadership positions (vice president of academic affairs, coach, teacher, fund-raiser, director of mental health clinic, etc.) due more to my enthusiasm and hard work than to my leadership qualities. I've never really been much of a leader except, in some cases, by example.

Finally, I never apologize for liking to make money and gain material goods—and then counting that money and admiring those material gains. It brings both satisfaction and security to me. I've made a lot of money in my life—and also given much of it away in a generous manner. Why should I deny this need in a free enterprise country when even many religious leaders (I could name them specifically) have amassed much material wealth and enjoy flaunting it. As mentioned previously, so does the institutional Catholic Church, 95% of protestant churches, and most of the world's other religions. So why shouldn't I—or you? Let's go get 'em!! I'll show you later that making money, in a free enterprise country, is so easy to do. IF YOU ARE A SUCCESS-ORIENTED PERSON, AND I'M ASSUMING YOU ARE, THE NEXT TWO CHAPTERS ALONE WILL BE WORTH THOUSANDS OF DOLLARS TO YOU! I would now give someone $80,000 if they would have taught me the next two chapters 25 years ago. I would have made it all back, plus much more, anyway.

The Walkian
Theory of Certain Success

The formula for success is very, very simple and easy. It is deciding that you TRULY, TRULY wish to put that formula into action that is difficult. Like most positive goals, most people just pay lip-service to high success. But they actually settle for low success rather than risk high failure. Following are my specific steps for certain success—completely detailed. As you lose weight and begin to take more and more pride in your appearance and life, the tri-lateral programming and "pills" will "mysteriously" lead you to success-type actions. I have kept all this so simple that I hope each one of you thinks when you're finished reading, "Gosh, I could have written that!" Then I'll know I've been successful. But, just as in part two, it is the EN-TIRE PACKAGE and putting it together and into action that counts.

A) WORK HARD

Need this one be explained too much? Nothing worthwhile is ever attained without effort and sweat of brow. In addition, every success in life—from love to money—has a price to pay and a risk to take. Though many people haven't learned so yet, there are few things in life as satisfying as a good hard day's work. I'm thankful that my family, both on my Mother's and Father's side, taught me this early. I still enjoy hard work and I still do it.

The first principle of any successful venture is "If it's going to get done, I've got to do it!" If it's going to happen, you've got to make it happen. No one else is going to do it for you—or make it happen for you. Only failure-type people think in this manner. In any culture, hard work is in some way rewarded and sluggishness (including over-sleeping) is somehow punished. Many people refute this by pointing to unionism, public schools and other forms of socialistic programs. But even in the cultures of socialism and com-munism, the hard workers and the cunning and creative rise to the top. THERE IS ALWAYS ROOM AT THE TOP—BUT SELDOM ROOM TO SIT DOWN! My Grandfather (the late and great O. R. Henry of Jackson, Ohio,) taught me that many years ago.

If I were king of the world, which I'm sure as heck not and sure as heck don't wish to be, the first decree I'd make is a flat-out law of NO WORKEE—NO EATEE! I'm dead serious and want to explain this so no one misunderstands me or my motives on this subject. NO WORKEE—NO EATEE, and there would be darn few exceptions. Only the completely, com-pletely elderly and infirm and only the entirely, entirely disabled.

In my world, no one would receive free lunches. That is, no one would get social, governmental monies (in essence, money from other working people) UNLESS they did something productive to help make the world better in some manner. Let me give you some extreme examples (which will probably anger many of you) and then permit me to attempt at least to justify my position:

A) There would be absolutely no A.D.C. and welfare checks handed out without productivity in return. As an elementary example, if there are three women with dependent children, one of the women would be expected to "babysit" for a month with the three childen while the other two went out and picked up litter, painted guard rails, mowed weeds, planted flowers in public parks, etc. The next month, the mothers would rotate duties. That simple. But they won't sit at home doing nothing and receive a check for eating chocolates, drinking beer, and watching General Hospital in my world. There's too much work to be done. And, as you'll see in a moment with all my examples, I have further motive.

B) A man with a "bad back" (I have one) will at least be expected to do whatever work he can in order to draw a disability check. Quite honestly, I see many of them every day hoisting motors out of cars, but even if their back is actually highly damaged, they would be expected to address envelopes for the state highway department—or some similar production—in order to receive their monthly check. These "bad back" guys are sure lucky I'm not their king.

C) But let's take some real extremes to see if I can make you all mad. What about a person in an iron lung? Well, IF he can learn to address envelopes with a pen in his teeth, and IF he has the energy to do same for 15 minutes per day, then he'll be expected to do just that in order to get his renumeration. IF he can't, of course, then he'll be one of the rare exceptions that we'll take care of. I am Christian and humane, you know. But there won't be many. For example, use your creativity, maybe that person can be productive by teaching others like him how to "talk" with their eyes. Now there would be a good job for him.

And finally, what about the wounded, paraplegic veteran in a wheelchair who has valiantly fought for his country and our freedoms. You are grateful to him and so, by golly, am I. How about him? Yep, you guessed it, he must produce, too. IF he can get out in his wheelchair for one hour per day and pick up a little litter here and there, or paint a section of guard rail, he'll be expected to do that in order to earn his daily bread.

I suppose that all of this, especially since I've listed extremes in order to make a point, sounds hard-hearted and calloused, doesn't it? Well, not really. You see, not only does society have much work to be done, but I'm also concerned with all these people's self-concept and self-worth. Almost everyone needs to feel that they are needed and worthy, and almost no one wishes to feel that they are a drain on family and society. Most want a chance to contribute and to have their place in the sun. And for those few who don't have such needs? Well, we'll give them ample opportunity to develop those values. And how about those "scrotes" who don't, you ask? Then they won't eat. It's that simple.

Funny, I've seldom met a politican who didn't agree with my stance when I confronted him with it in private. But when it comes time to vote in such legislation and vote out all the give-away programs, we have become such a socialistic nation that he simply votes the way all his social program constituents want him to in order to keep his plush job. And then we wonder why we have a huge budget deficit. A tragedy!

B) PLAY HARD

But "Pop" Henry forgot to teach me something else important—probably because he'd never learned it himself. Therefore, he couldn't teach it to the rest of his family. So, few of them practice it. And I had to learn it the HARD way, unfortunately. That is, YOU MUST ALSO PLAY HARD! You must search for enjoyable relaxation of stress just as diligently as you seek achievement. If not, you either "break" in some manner or another and/or your successes become shallow and insignificant. I work hard—but I play hard. If I marry again, I'll do so early in the morning—so if it doesn't work out it won't ruin my whole day! Ha!

I take pride in conscientious work habits (I average five to six hours sleep per night), but I am equally proud of my "play" lifestyle. When I party, I party "hearty," and no one need try to make me feel guilty about doing so—though many have tried, from my Mother to church-goers, and from school newspaper writers to moralistic do-gooders. So long as I hurt no one else, my private life in a free country is mine—and mine alone. I'll do with it what I like, Mommy, reverend, boss, newspaper editors, police, and other authority figures. Any of you readers out there want to play and party? Call me anytime—except when I'm working! By the way, "partying" does not necessarily mean drugs or alcohol. I do NO drugs and now drink very sparingly. To plays means to have fun with no further purpose.

By the way, I've found over the years that the persons who detest my "play" most are wives of my male friends. Doggedly they work to keep their husbands away from the big, bad wolf (Walke) and at home on the leash. They are so fearful that the Walke-man will lead their "loyal old dogs" astray. Interestingly, 95% of my play is clean fun (that leaves 5% for INTRIGUE) and it is usually their confined husand who takes the LEAD when we socialize to STRAY into those "intriguing" areas. When, oh when, will women learn about men? And vice versa for all you feminist readers. Alas, the battle of the sexes rages eternally!

I had to learn the hard way about the importance of play. I was a workaholic from 13 years old until 35. I accomplished and achieved much, but was so driven that those, the prime years of my life, were basically unhappy, burdensome, painful years. I'll always regret that, and I'll never be able to recapture those years, but I'll never make that mistake again. Don't you either!

DREAM YOUR DREAMS AND WORK HARD/PLAY HARD TO MAKE THEM COME TRUE

I have been asked many times what I think is the true meaning of life or what I think the major goal of life should be. Well, obviously the answer is "I don't really know—those questions have different answers for different people." Some people would answer them in a very religious way, believing that the whole significance of life on this planet is to prepare for another life yet to come in another setting—heaven, land of the setting sun, happy hunting ground, shangri-la, etc. They may well be correct and I respect their views. I honestly hope that they are right in their beliefs.

Other people would feel that love and our relationships with other human beings and animals are "where it's at." To those people, the need to love and be loved is the center of the cosmos. They would feel—as all humanists do—that man's humanity to man overshadows all else and that any other purpose pales in its presence. I also would not find any argument with this point-of-view because no matter what one gains in his short stay on this earth, those "honors" would be empty without the "sharing-ness" of them with allied others—people with whom we AFFILIATE in various depths of feeling. Howard Hughes proved that loudly and clearly.

Therefore, I will concede the two life-approaches above and plead "no contest." But there is another viewpoint that goes hand-in-hand that both moralists and humanists must also concede because MOST of them practice it whether they know it or not—or whether they admit it or not, that is, that the only true significance of life on this spheroid is to DREAM YOUR DREAMS AND THEN TO WORK HARD (AND PLAY HARD) TO MAKE THEM COME TRUE! I just flat-out don't know of anything else—already having conceded the previous two. What else is there? I absolutely and positively can't think of anything. If you know of anything more meaningful, would you please let me know?

All of you know of many people who work very, very hard all of their lives but who just don't seem to ever formulate any large scale dreams or goals. You probably also know of myriads of humans who dream and fantasize all the time but never carry-out plans to bring them to fruition. Both groups squander their brief lives serving as talkers—not doers. There is no need to criticize them because they constitute the vast majority and one can argue that "they are just as good as anyone else"—which is obviously true.

But I contend that there is a small group of earth inhabitants who live beyond the "common herd." That select group of homo sapiens is those who do not base any part of their life on memories—just on dreams. They continually dream their dreams and set high goals and then continually work hard to make them all come to pass—remembering how to play along the way. They see life as a continual process of growth and development.

Maslow called these people SELF-ACTUALIZED! That's a very good description. Others call it "becoming more fully human." That's nice, too. I just like to call it "rising above the common herd." Only a very elite group is willing and able to do it. Why not you? It's just as easy as the lifestyle you've been taught.

C) GOOD HUMAN RELATIONS SKILLS

Just as weight loss-weight control is a specialized area for me, so is self-concept (to be discussed soon) and human relations skills. Please note at this point that the heading above does NOT say PUBLIC relations skills—but HUMAN relations skills. What we will be discussing here is how one human being relates to another human being in a genuine, sincere manner—on a one-to-one basis. We will not be discussing how a company relates to the masses; or how a corporation covers up its malpractices, or an individual who is a "back-slapper" who is only nice to you because he hopes to sell you a car, sweeper, or insurance policy in the near future. Aren't those false "game players" despicable—and obnoxious, and boring, and ad infinitum? There is little worse in this world than a person who feigns (fakes) affection simply for "PR" reasons. I am convinced that we humans can somehow sense (vibes?) sincere emotional affection or lack of same and therefore resent false "PR" people.

"There are, in my opinion, eight basic human relation skills. I've held seminars detailing them all over the midwest and will do so for you here now. I'm quite proud of what I'm about to present to you. It is a classic example of simplicity, but if you put the entire package to work for you, you'll be highly successful and/or make a lot of money. IT IS MY EXPERIENCE THAT ONLY ABOUT .01% OF OUR POPULATION POSSESS ALL EIGHT OF THESE SKILLS AND THAT THOSE PERSONS ARE

ALWAYS AS SUCCESSFUL AS THEY WISH TO BE!!! For example then, if you live in a community with 30,000 people, only about 30 people have ALL EIGHT skills, and whether they be butcher, baker, candlestick-maker, housewife, banker, corporation president or whatever, they will most always be successful in whatever manner they define it. If you hail from a community of 8,000, as I do, then only approximately eight people possess and practice all eight of the skills. So if you develop them, you automatically become a part of a very elite group. Just think, a city of one million only has 1,000 such persons.

I've never thought it was mere coincidence that the man who is the most successful man in our county—by most standards of success—is the man who best practices ALL EIGHT of these skills. In fact, he is a master of them in his daily life. Little wonder that he is a highly popular and successful businessman; that he has also reigned longer than anyone else in Ohio's history as the Speaker of the House; and that he may well be over-all the most powerful and prestigious man in Ohio. I speak, of course, of the aforementioned Honorable Vernal G. Riffe. Watching him deftly practice my eight human relation skills is like watching a skilled brain surgeon at work! And any of you can do the same if you TRULY wish to do so. Permit me to show you how. I like to shock my classes by picking out any reasonably attractive woman or man and show them how they can be the governor of Ohio within 20 years and that even if they don't make it, they'll still be highly successful and will have had a lot of fun and challenge along the way.

1) EYE CONTACT-TACTILE CONTACT

Check something for yourself. Tally how few people make direct and in-timate eye contact with you during your daily life except A) to show aggres-sion towards you (stare you down) or B) to make sexual contact (make eyes at you or, if you please, "make out with you"). Other than these two excep-tions, seldom will another person relate to you in a sincere, genuine manner through direct eye contact. Instead, they will either look through you, look upward and downward, or focus on a point past your shoulder.

Yet, one of the major ways we humans relate to one another in a "love ac-tion" way is to intimately confront each other with our eyes. And as we make eye contact with others, we are drawing those persons into us—making them a part of us, WHETHER OR NOT THEY REALIZE IT. In essence, you are inviting them into your life and you are becoming a part of theirs. All this occurs automatically (and unconsciously) and neither they nor you can prevent it.

I cannot prove what I'm about to present to you, but there is absolutely no doubt in my mind that I'm correct. Let's pretend that we had a barometer which would exactly measure how much one human being likes or dislikes another. Let's further say that it registers that you dislike me 99.67% (wow, what on earth did I do to you?). Let's now hypothesize that each time I encounter you I make direct eye contact. Even if I don't say a word to you, I'll bet you $1,000 that after a short period of time, the barometer reading would at least go down to 99.66% and, in all probability, much further. Eye contact is a very personal and powerful instrument.

Such a small percentage of humans are capable of making these brief—but effective—eye contacts on a daily basis (even with strangers) that you are already becoming a part of a very elite group. We have already gone from 100% down to probably 5% in our quest for the final .01% club.

By developing your self-concept, and therefore your ability to draw people nearer to you through eye contact, you are taking a giant step toward effective human relations. Let's hypothesize that you would tell me you're presently a lonely person with few friends. If you begin to make sincere eye contact with, let's say, approximately 100 persons per day (don't laboriously keep count, for goodness sake), I wager you'll find yourself SOON being less lonely and possessing more friends—at least platonic ones. Eyes are psychological magnets, and they will polarize people in your direction over a period of time. Try it.

Let's further hypothesize that you tell me that you're not as effective in your salesmanship as you might like. Make 100 eye contacts per day (700 genuine eye contacts per week, 5,200 annually, 52,000 in a short decade), and watch your sales jump over a period of a few weeks or months. Eye contact is a magical tool for cementing relationships. There may be successful people who don't possess this skill, but rarely is there a person who possesses the skill who isn't at least BEGINNING to find success. Humans desperately need "love actions" and they will consciously or unconsciously work FOR the person who gives those actions to them and against those who don't. I am convinced this is a universal truth. People will actually labor to make you successful if you continually and genuinely eye contact them.

The same is true of tactile contact (touching). Touching is equally as effective as a "love action" between humans. Yet, isn't it amazing how many people seem incapable of warm touching of others or of being warmly touched? How many of us can observe that even our own parents rarely, if ever, touched us in any way except maybe to spank us. Hard to believe, isn't it? It is also easily discernible how many people do not like to be touched and even feel threatened by it. Yet, I contend, they are at least subliminally liking it and responding positively to a sincere touch.

I have never thought the bumper sticker "Have You Hugged Your Child Today?" was completely necessary. "Have You Touched Your Child Today?" is just as relevant since any type of light touch—i. e., hand on shoulder, finger on nose or face, tousling of hair, etc.—is an act of love, if done sincerely.

I might add that hard back slapping (or butt), pinching, etc. are acts of latent aggression and are not related. When a person slaps you hard on the back and says, "Glad to see you!," he isn't glad to see you at all and is showing so by his actions. He is displaying aggressive hostility and resentment toward you, though he may not realize it himself. And though he may rationalize that he "doesn't know his own strength," he can be reminded that even the biggest, strongest gorilla/ape can lay his hand lightly on another's back or hold a peanut in its hand without crushing it.

In any event, learn to reach out and touch others. Aha, be an A. T. & T. person! Because, touching also invites people into your life—and they like that. I mentioned salesmen a moment ago. Ironically, most salesmen are backslappers, for whatever reason. If they would just learn to be "touchers," their commissions would increase significantly—all else being equal. A recent legitimate study proved that even waitresses who lightly touch patrons when presenting the check will receive over-all better tips than those who don't.

SPECIAL NOTE:

Obviously, too much of a good thing is harmful. One cannot go around making eye contact with EVERYONE and touching EVERYONE. Heaven forbid! But so long as your sensory contact is genuine, it would be difficult to OVER-DO IT.

So, let's just suppose that you purposely made eye contact with 700 persons per week and tactile contact with the same number. That's 1,400 per week, 72,800 per year, 728,000 in a brief decade. Wow, your "outreach" to other humans within five or ten years would be astronomical, as would the beginning of your success. And we're only finalizing ONE skill. We have seven to go. If you are a consistent eye-contactor and toucher, you're probably already in the 4% club. But we're headed for the .01% club.

I know a politician right now who has achieved many re-elections just on the ability to shake hands and remember names alone. He has few other abilities. And even his genuineness and credibility are questionable. But he boasts that he's shaken hands with more people than anyone else in Ohio—and he probably has. So, just think of what you can accomplish with what we are about to learn!

2) A FIRM HAND SHAKE (COMBINED WITH EYE CONTACT)

The percentage of people who are quality hand-shakers is also very small. Seldom do you meet a person who is really competent in this skill. Most will have at least one (or more) of the following weaknesses:

A) They simply do not shake hands at all due either to shyness (poor self-concept), arrogance and aloofness, or lack of social knowledge or skills.

B) They extend a weak, limp hand shake with dropped eyes—again due to shyness and negative self-image.

C) They give a weak, limp hand to you while looking through you or above you as a sign of contempt for or aloofness from you.

D) They shake hands competitively (usually men) and in a macho manner—using the ritual as a test of strength and/or endurance. These men usually possess a deep need to continually prove their manhood and the hand shake is one of latent aggression, designed to overcome you. There is little sincereity or genuineness involved. People quickly (again, usually unconsciously) work "against" their success.

E) Hand shake hesitancy. People are not certain if they wish to shake hands with another or if they SHOULD do so either due to the social situation or sexual difference.

SPECIAL NOTE TO WOMEN

Here's an excellent tip to women who wish to be successful. I have noted that most women are hesitant to INITIATE a hand shake—especially with men and quite often even with other women. This is especially true during our present "transition" period into womens' rights. However, it is completely socially-acceptable for you to initiate a hand shake—and, in fact, I contend that it is a very good idea. Not only does it naturally draw people to you, but it takes the pressure off the male—who also usually is not certain (during this transition period) whether he should originate the hand shake with a woman. Therefore, women who take a hand shaking initiative are already a step ahead of fellow women—and many men—in ventures toward success.

So, as you develop the skill to shake hands sincerely—combined with eye and tactile contact (i.e., placing the other hand lightly on another's hand, arm or shoulder)—you gain tremendous ability to reach out to others and draw them into you. Again, even though they may not realize it, you are "taking them into your life."

People with excellent human relation skills who also have high achievement and success needs should practice skills #1 and #2 profusely—without running them into the ground. For example, do not hesitate a moment to shake hands with even a close friend on a reasonably periodic basis (perhaps once weekly). And fear not to shake hands with new acquaintances or even strangers. Whatever your definition of success, watch it begin to happen! Just look at pure mathematics. You shake hands with approximately 100 persons per day; at least make eye contact with 100; and eye contact and touch another 100. 300 per day, 2,100 per week, 109,200 contacts per year, 1,092,000 in a decade. You're flat-out relating now, my friend, and wait until I show you the many, many ways it will help you. I'm hoping to "blow your mind." Let us continue.

3) PAYING A SINCERE COMPLIMENT

I have long been a greater believer in flowers for the living and not the dead. How depressing it is that most human beings go through life unable to pay a sincere compliment or praise another human, yet then go through the silly, guilt-easing ritual of buying flower wreaths for that same person after he has died. Gamesmanship at its ultimate height—and most morbid low.

The past year I've lost two of the dearest people in my life—my Father and my favorite Uncle, Ed Henry. How thankful I am that many times I told my Father what a good man he was (in various ways) and how much he meant to me. I even went so far as to write an open tribute to my Dad's positive attributes and had it published into a wall poster with a 43-year-old picture of my youthful Father and me as a three-year-old boy in the poster background. It was presented to Dad long before he died. He loved it—and cried, which I seldom saw him do. No funeral flowers—which die quickly—were necessary. In my opinion, they seldom are—except as a public relations instrument or guilt-ridding tool. Send me flowers and/or pay me compliments while I'm alive. I could care less, or know less, after I pass away. I wrote my uncle on various occasions and outlined specifically why he had always been my favorite uncle and why I thought he was such a great man. Those letters meant much more to him than roses, mums or geraniums, and they certainly meant more to HIM than the hundreds of funeral wreaths he received.

Very few people, percentage-wise, are able to pay compliments to others. It is related, of course, to egocentricism and the fact that most people are just too "sensititve" (lack of ego strength) to tell others that "you look nice;" "that's a pretty blouse;" "man, you played a great game last night," etc. My father, excellent man that he was, was seldom able to compliment me and I so yearned for it, as most children do. He would boast to others about me but just didn't have the nerve (ability) to tell me.

I tell my students, IF you think I'm a good teacher or even a great teacher, tell me so soon. Don't wait until I die of a heart attack or cancer and then sing my praises (eulogize). I won't give a darn then but now it would mean EVERYTHING to me—as it would most teachers. We sure as heck ain't in it for the money!

When you pay sincere compliments to people, even though they may be a little embarrassed at the moment, they are pleased and you are becoming a part of their life—and they, yours. You can put them to work for you some-day IF your compliment was genuine. Go to the bank on it!

I pay a lot of compliments to people—even complete strangers. With women, it's quite easy to get branded as a "flirt" and with men as a "bullshitter" if you do not follow one ground-rule very religiously:

NEVER PAY ANYONE A COMPLIMENT
UNLESS YOU TRULY FEEL IT AND MEAN IT!!!

Gamesmanship is bad enough, anyway. But it becomes atrocious if you play games with your compliments. I'm firmly convinced that we humans can actually sense sincere compliments versus false compliments. I further believe we'll soon be able to scientifically prove I'm right through the use of pupillametrics. In the meantime, don't say it if you don't mean it. Inversely, if you DO feel it and mean it—for GOD'S sake, SAY IT! You'll bind people to you in droves. People love to be "stroked"—if it's sincere. Though they may appear—and actually be—embarrassed, they will magnetically be drawn to you. It's a universal law!

Now, you see, these first three skills become cumulative (that is, like a snowball going down a hill). When you put all three together, and practice them daily and "promiscuously," you'll soon be relating to so many humans and so many humans will be in turn relating to you. Hence, human relations skills! Already, after covering only three of eight skills, we're down to possibly three percent of the population, and probably less. Very few people you meet possess and practice just these three simple principles. Their lack of growth and development prevents it. Just look at how you'll soon be part of the "cream" which rises to the top. And you will rise to the top in many ways.

4) ACKNOWLEDGING A COMPLIMENT

Whew, this one was the toughest for me of all eight. I think the same is true of most of us. When one says something complimentary to us, our egocentricism seems to switch into high gear. We become flustered and either try to act humble and/or pretend it wasn't stated, and thus, "scuff it off"—even though we adore hearing those positive words. So, we usually discover ourselves saying something like "Oh, it's nothing" or "Aw, it's not much" while we drop our eyes in mock humility. I say "mock" because, if we're honest, we not only thought we deserved the compliment—but sought it, either by the way we dressed; the feat we accomplished; the gem of wisdom we stated; or that which we created.

It took me many years to develop the proper presence—when someone said, "Dr. Walke, you are an excellent teacher and have helped my life so much"—to reply (while making eye contact and usually shaking hands) "Thank you, it means a lot to me that you feel that way. By the way, you also have been a very conscientious student!" (If I mean it). Do you realize that I have just exhibited all four of the human relation skills discussed thus far and cemented that person's relationship forever! That person will consciously and/or unconsciously work toward my success so long as I live on this earth—assuming everything I did was sincere. Are you beginning—just beginning—to see how easy it all is? And we're only half way home! And you're probably already down to at least the 2% club, possibly lower. Let us proceed. But begin to practice and develop these four skills immediately. And make no mistake, they can be developed!

5) COMMON COURTESY

The Golden Rule is so simple. Then why do I encounter so many people who do not practice it? You meet them all the time, too, don't you? So did Jesus! How many of us treat MOST people MOST of the time as we would like to be treated in that situation? Common courtesy—at the supermarket, the department store, on the job, in church, at school—is so difficult to find. I HAVE FOUND THAT EVEN COLLEGE FACULTY, SUPPOSEDLY THE MOST ENLIGHTENED OF OUR SOCIETY, SELDOM PRACTICE IT! We are all so entangled in our own biases, jealousies and envies, and personal needs, that we just cannot treat people as we would expect to be treated. That's why we get branded as LITTLE PEOPLE! Only a few of my colleagues at Shawnee State are BIG PEOPLE—persons who practice common courtesy and the Golden Rule—and they are so refreshing. The remainder live small lives—and they'll never know large scale success, simply because they have few human relations' skills and are curt and rude unnecessarily to so many people. Their major goal seems to be just to exist—and to rain on others' parades. They'd rather sink the ship than have it sail without them.

I simply do not think that way. I attempt to continually take the approach: "I'm interested in your success, not your failure!" Let's all be successful. Me, of course! But all of you, too! Why is life so full of the little people? "Scorpions" multiply easily, I guess. And, of course, we're back to self-concept problems again.

6) CREATIVE LISTENING

You probably realize that very few people (percentage-wise) are good, attentive listeners. Listening is still another form of sensory contact and one of the major actions of love we show to others is to LISTEN to them. I have often said that a parent who seldom listens to his/her children is already proving a very limited depth of love for that child. The same is true in relating to any other person. If you do not listen, your relationship with them is shallow at most. No matter how much you tell someone you love them, if you make little sensory contact with them and do not listen to them, the depth of that relationship is highly limited. But further note that I've used the term CREATIVE listening. What does that mean? In psychology and counseling, a word that has become most "shopworn" is the word EMPATHETIC. Nevertheless, it is a good word—meaning to try to the utmost to place yourself in anothers' shoes (head) and to think what he is thinking and feel what he is feeling. Of course, to accomplish this ENTIRELY is impossible. For me to ever say that I know what it's like to be a woman, or Black, or Jewish, or German would be ludicrous and presumptuous.

But by creatively listening to another, we can EMPATHIZE with them—that is, to come as close as it is possible to come to crawling inside their mind and feel what they are feeling and think what they are thinking.

The major tool of creative listening is REFLECTION. With the careful and prudent use of reflection, you cannot only listen to the words and phrases of another, but you can "draw him out" and have him define his terms and feelings in the manner he is stating them to you. Let me give you a few examples:

A) A friend says to you, "My wife and I are getting along terribly." Now you know what the word "terribly" means to you, but you don't know in what context HE is using it. At this pont, you don't know what TERRIBLY means to him. If you are a good "human relater," you WANT to know. So, you make eye contact with him and simply state, "Terribly?" You do this in a sincere voice with upward inflection, so that he'll elaborate.

B) Let's say he answers, "Yes, terribly, we just don't seem to communicate." Again, you know how you define "communicate," but you don't know how he does. So you might respond "You don't communicate very well?'' (Upward voice inflection.)

C) Let's say he then states forlornly, ''No, we don't. She seldom talks to me while I'm home; she won't go places with me; she won't even come in and watch TV with me; she just wants me to be the loyal old dog around the house. I'm lonely in my own home!

D) You: ''Lonely?''

He: ''Yes, my own children don't talk to me either. It just seems they expect me to be there, yet I'm alone within the confines of my own walls.''

Now you know what he meant by ''Terribly!'' IF you had not used reflections, YOU might have thought he meant that she beat him, or cursed him, or berated him in front of others, etc. You can now begin to EMPATHIZE—rather than just sympathize—with this man. Therefore, once again, you are relating to him and drawing closer to him, and inviting him into you. So, however you define success, he'll probably begin to work for your success. Whether that's simply being a friend and providing companionship; buying a sweeper from you; voting for you in the next election; buying stock in a business venture you've created; or whatever. SEE HOW EASY IT IS TO BE SUCCESSFUL?

And I will assure you that we're already easily down to ONE PERCENT. Yes, only one percent of our population possess and daily practice ALL SIX of the above skills. You can therefore be part of a very ELITE group. But, we're not finished yet. Now, we will use skills #1 through #6 to devleop #7 and #8. Then you'll be ready to ''conquer the world'' (be successful) in any form you desire. OH, HOW I WISH SOMEONE WOULD HAVE TAUGHT ME ALL THIS WHEN I WAS 21! As I said previously, I would gladly have gone to the bank and borrowed $80,000 and paid it to them and then simply made monthly payments on it—because I would have made that $80,000 back so easily, plus much, much more.

7) MAKE CONTACTS (GET OUT AMONGST 'EM)

Even if you KNOW in your mind that you have the ability to practice human relations skills #1 through #6, it means ABSOLUTELY NOTHING unless you get out ''AMONGST 'EM'' and do it! You must be willing to use the first six skills to CONTINUALLY MAKE NEW HUMAN CONTACTS. The first six skills tell you HOW it is done—the final two explain what must be accomplished if you are to be successful.

Skill #7 (plus #8) have been commonly labeled over many years as ''KNOWING THE TERRITORY!'' And rightfully so. Rarely in an over-populated world can you be successful in any manner without the active aid of others. Sure, you can point to exceptions within creative fields of art, music, invention, science, etc. But you can't point out many! There are too many great minds today. You need help. And, even rarer still is the highly creative person who does seemingly accomplish greatness yet ENJOYS those accomplishments IF he has no human relations abilities. Successful, but tragic, schizoid personalities (deep fear of human relationships) are a dime a dozen. They are buried in ornate, yet lonely, mausoleums all over the globe. As far as I'm concerned, when Howard Hughes lost his human relations abilities, he died psychologically, even though he lived physically for many more years.

THE
KROGER'S SUPERMARKET PARABLE

I am going to relate to you one parable of making contacts. You can relate it to ANY and EVERY situation you wish. It always applies. Let's hypothesize that both you and I possess skills #1 - #6 and that we both go to a Kroger's supermarket and purchase a great steak which is super tender and melts in our mouth as we consume it. Our guests at our cook-out are also much impressed.

However, there is one major difference between you and me. It seems reasonable, all other things being equal, that we'll both continue to shop at Kroger's in the near future—at least when it comes time to shop for steak. So, let us say we both return to Kroger's the week following (remember that we both possess human relations skills #1 - #6 equally). You purchase your meat, possibly tell the check-out person you've seen previously how attractive her blouse is (if you mean it), and head for home. However, I'm going to spend maybe five minutes more in Kroger's than you. Just five little minutes—because I know that when push comes to shove, all I really have in life is TIME, only an explicit amount of time. So, I stop by the store manager's office (let's call him Mr. Jones since that's what the office door nameplate reads).

Utilizing all six skills above, I state (while shaking hands and making eye contact), "Mr. Jones, my name is Jerry Walke. I teach down at Shawnee State College. I just wanted to tell you that last week I purchased here what perhaps was the best piece of steak I've ever tasted in my life. It literally melted in my mouth! And my cook-out guests also enjoyed it immensely."

I don't know how well developed are the human relations skills of Mr. Jones. But let's again hypothesize that he replies, "Thank you, Mr. Walke.

We like to hear those things. By the way, our head meatcutter, Mr. Smith works behind the scenes most of the time and doesn't get much credit for his fine work. You might want to stop back and tell him what you just told me."

"Thank you Mr. Jones, I'll make a point to see him right now," I respond.

I quickly walk to the "Employee's Only" door in the rear—which I've just been given permission to enter. I approach Mr. Smith, make eye contact, firmly shake his hand, and say sincerely, "Mr. Smith, my name is Jerry Walke. I'm a teacher down at the college. I just told Mr. Jones (now I just used public relations, not human relations—letting him know I complimented him to his boss) that last week I bought here what was perhaps the best steak I've ever eaten. You can be proud of that quality of cut."

Eyes beaming, Mr. Smith replies, "Thank you Mr. Walke, I don't get many compliments like that here in the backroom."

"You're welcome, Bill (on his name tag), keep up the good work." I then head for home—possibly telling the check-out person on the way out that her blouse is very attractive—assuming I also think it is.

Now you may be saying "So what?" What do you mean "So what?" I'll SHOW you "So what?" Let's again hypothesize that I meet FOUR new people each day—make four NEW CONTACTS each day—in the same manner (which I will) and that you don't. That tallies up to 28 more people per week that I know that you don't know. That computes to 126 per month of people I have confronted and "eyeballed" personally that you haven't. This builds into 1,512 annually and 15,120 over a short, quick decade. Also keep in mind that MOST of those people will tell at LEAST one other person—even if a spouse, his/her children, etc.—both about me and the compliment. It is reasonable to assume that Jerry Walke will be perceived in a positive manner by approximately 30,000 more people (quite frankly, it will probably be many more) who will consciously and/or unconsciously work for my success. Then add that figure to my previous statistics on skills #1, #2, and #3. Look out world, here I (you) come!

WELCOME TO THE SCIENTIFIC AGE

But how are you going to use all those staggering statistics you are gathering to your benefit? Well, the sky (actually, your own creativity) is the limit. I'll provide you some further insights after we discuss skill #8, but in the meantime let me give you a tip worth far more than you'll ever pay for this book. Oh, how I wish someone would have impressed this one on me 25 years ago. I just started it five years ago and I can't believe the results. I literally get tears in my eyes thinking what would have happened had I started this at 21.

You see, if the opportunity presents itself, I will ask Mr. Jones and Mr. Smith for their business card. If they do not have one, or if the "common courtesy" situation isn't right to inquire of them (i.e., they're too busy), I'll do some investigative work (telephone book, asking around, etc.) and get their complete home address and phone—or at least their business address and phone. Then that evening (or sometime soon), I enter that information in my home computer—and I cross-reference it. So, at any time, just by pushing a few code keys, I can get a complete print-out of all personal contacts I know in Portsmouth, Cincinnati, Philadelphia, etc. But I can also get a print-out of all grocery store managers, meat cutters, ministers, school administrators, coaches, etc. with whom I've had personal contacts. Or I can simply get a complete ALPHABETIZED list of contacts for mass mailing or phoning. Or a print-out of all people in Ohio; or a alphabetized list of meat cutters in Ohio, etc., ad in finitum. Starting to get the picture? Wait until I show you possible ways you can utilize this later.

8) "MENDING FENCES" (MAINTAINING CONTACTS)

Let's now go back to Kroger's parable for scene two. Once you have related to a new person in an atmosphere of sincerity, it is very satisfying (and wise) to continue that relationship. Perhaps it will become a fairly intimate one, or what we call a lasting friendship. Naturally, more often than not, it will be on a more superficial basis—but still positive and wholesome.

For example, let's now create a scenario six weeks after the complimentary exchange at Kroger's. Let's say that I've had another truly nice experience at Kroger's—the produce manager selected for me a succulent watermelon. I not only pay him the compliment (new contact) but drop by the manager's office again. "Mr. Jones, you may not remember me, but I'm Jerry Walke from the college."

"Oh yes, Mr. Walke. I remember you and that you stopped by to tell us nice things about our meat department. You know, Mr. Smith was very pleased."

"Thank you. Well, I stopped by this time to say that Mr. Fritz, your produce manager, recently took the time to select an excellent watermelon for a party I was having. My guests loved it. I really appreciated his doing that—and am so impressed with how he relates to customers (if I mean it). I just told him so."

"Well, thank you again, Mr. Walke. We're happy you like our store and service."

"Yes, I do. By the way, do you have a business card? The vice-president for advertising of your company is a friend of mine. We went from kindergarten through college together. (By the way, that is absolutely true. John Richard Owens is his name). I'm going to drop him a note about the excellence of this store." (If Mr. Jones isn't pleased with THAT jesture, then he isn't a member of the human race).

I then take a minute or so to stop by the meat department. "Mr. Smith, do you remember me? Jerry Walke."

"Yes, Mr. Walke I certainly do! You got one of our mouth-watering steaks."

"Yes, I just wanted to stop by and say hello. How are things going? (We then may converse, but I'll leave the amount of talking to him so as not to be obnoxious—common courtesy, skill #5. Remember)?

So, you see, today I spent five minutes, made another new contact, and further cemented two previous ones. Watch what may well come of all this in the future. Willie Nelson says, "What goes 'round comes 'round," AND THAT IS CERTAINLY A UNIVERSAL TRUTH! Whether your actions be positive, negative, or non-existent, they will come back to help you or haunt you. I've been down both those roads.

A "TIP" FOR YOU
EASILY WORTH THE PRICE OF
THIS BOOK

Let me further elaborate now on my discussion two pages back. I DID ask for Mr. Jones business card in order to write the letter to the Kroger executive. Don't play games with people. You eventually get caught. I have and so have you. But I also did so because, when I get home, I'll enter Mr. Jones complete name, address, and phone number to my list of contacts and mailing list. As mentioned, I now keep such a list and it is extensive—cross indexed by city, state, and the person's profession. It is so easy to do all this in our modern age of word processors and home computers. I'll also look-up Mr. Smith and Mr. Fritz's names and addresses in the phone book and record them.

You should see my list—enhanced even more by each and every one of my students the past five years. If only I would have started this practice when I began my teaching TWENTY-FIVE years ago. My list would be flat-out AWESOME! The uses of such a list are limited only by your imagination and creativity—as well as by your definition of success.

A simple example of how you might use these personal contacts. You receive much junk mail, do you not? And MOST of you, like me, immediately toss MOST of it into file 13 (the waste basket), right? HOWEVER, if the inside address contains the name of someone you know or have met personally, you'll AT LEAST open it. Correct?

And even though you may not decide to act upon whatever is inside because it has no interest to you, it is proven that a given percentage of people will respond, both because what inside does have interest to them (let's say something simple—like the sale of Christmas cards) or because they know the person. You see, they've probably already thrown away three other "junk mailers" advertising Christmas cards without even opening them.

So, if you're into Christmas cards (which I'm not), I'll profit a few thousand dollars at Christmas time while you frustratingly make $169.00 and don't even cover your postage—and give up—SIMPLY BECAUSE YOU DON'T USE SKILLS #1 - #6 TO DEVELOP #7 AND #8. YOU JUST DON'T KNOW THE TERRITORY! You avoided making and maintaining contacts with the Mr. Jones', Mr. Smiths' and Mr. Fritzs'—and thousands of others. I spent a little extra time in Kroger's using my human relations skills while you hustled home to watch the ballgame. Interestingly, I also watched that game while you wasted five minutes waiting for it to come on. Remember the old bull—young bull story?

BUT LOOK WHAT HAPPENS NEXT!

About now you may be thinking, "Well, I'm not into Christmas cards, or selling books, or country music tapes, or widgets, or whatever, by mail. Fine, but let's look further, Let's speculate that it's now two years later. Your wife has applied for the only vacant position at a local school and so has mine. And, for the sake of argument, let's further say that they are completely equal in credentials, transcripts, attractiveness and grooming, articulateness, recommendations, etc. In competiveness, you must always assume that all other factors are equal and seek "THE EDGE."

But, low and behold, guess who we find is the local school board president? You guessed it, Mr. Jones, the manager of Kroger's. All else being equal, remember, you and your wife will never even know what hit you. My wife will, in all probability, be teaching at Midvale Elementary next year while yours, devastated, sits at home or takes a job which isn't as fulfilling to her.

And you can cry out "politics" or whatever you wish. That's the way the world works, isn't it? All else being equal, what would you have done in Mr. Jones's position, flip a coin? No, you would have done just what he did—either consciously or UNCONSCIOUSLY: You would have subliminally "Halo effected" Mrs. Walke because of Mr. Walke's human relations skills. Now your home is not quite as serene as mine is, all because you couldn't or wouldn't spend a few extra minutes in Kroger's exercising your human relation skills. You don't know the territory, boy!

But it gets worse. Your daughter has just graduated as a registered nurse. So has mine. Your daughter has just applied for the vacant position as city health nurse and so has mine. Again, assume they are completely equal in training, degrees, personal appearance, bedside manner, etc. The job is a prestigious "plum" that they both want badly since they are young and will have to work the midnight shift if they go into the local hospital. Assume further they are the only two applicants—just to make the point.

But wonder of all wonders, guess who the president of city council is? Yes, you guessed it again, Mr. Smith, the head meat cutter at Krogers. All else being equal, my man, your daughter will be working midnight shift at the hospital while struggling to make a success of her new marriage while my daughter contentedly fulfills her duties as city health nurse with nice daytime hours and weekends off with her new husband. "Sorry Charlie!" You snooze, you lose! Actually, I used this parable on purpose. Many of you are probably thinking its quite far-fetched. Not at all. A few years ago—in my hometown—the local supermarket manager was president of the school board and the head meat-cutter was president of the city council. Back to Willie Nelson and his insightful statement, "What goes 'round, comes 'round." It's a universal truth. And when you use all eight human relations skills on a daily basis, it will always come back around to lift you to almost any success you desire. I repeat, at most .01% of our population practice all eight, and they are almost without exception as successful as they wish to be. Especially when you combine all eight with hard work; hard play; and what follows in Chapter Thirteen.

IN AMERICA,
MAKING MONEY IS SO EASY!

We're not even close to finished with the Walkian Formula for certain success yet, but let's take a "time out" to discuss some specifics of how the eight human relations skills can be effectively utilized to make monetary profits— just in case that is YOUR definition of success. Making bucks is as easy as falling off a log if you practice just hard work, hard play, and wholesome human relations. Then the next chapter will show you how to make BIG BUCKS!

I've already shown you how to make profits from junk mail (or phone sales) of Christmas cards or whatever half-way useful product you wish to sell. But let me give you further uses and let's start out with some outlandish ones just to make the point.

A) FREDDIE, THE FREELOADER

Your moral and ethical fabric would probably not allow you to do this—and neither would mine. I carry my own load wherever I go and take pride in doing so—as I'm sure you do. But simply for the sake of bringing home my point, let's say that right now I was broke, yet wanted to take a year off from my job and VACATION all over the U.S.A. Could I do it? You bet your buttocks I can—me and my little home computer. Simply because I have worked hard and developed and used my human relations skills.

I can sit down right now at my console and plan a year-long itinerary to Cincinnati, Columbus, Cleveland, Detroit, Chicago, New York, Philadelphia, Boston, Tampa, Orlando, Beloxi, New Orleans, Houston, Dallas, Tucson, Phoenix, Colorado Springs, Las Vegas, San Diego, Los Angeles, San Francisco, Seattle, Salt Lake City, Minneapolis, St. Louis, and back home. There are many other cities I haven't named. In each city, I assure you that there are people who will be happy to have me as their guest—room and board free for at least a week, and they probably won't let me buy anything while I'm there if I don't wish to. All from just "knowing the territory."

B) OUTRIGHT BUMMING

How about an even more shocking example—and another one which my "up-bringing" would not allow me to do without much guilt. What if I were flat-broke right now and told you that one month from now I could retire with $100,000 cash, go to Florida or California and draw $1,000 Dollars per month, just in interest (based on prime rates at time of writing this book) the reminder of my life.

Far-fetched? Nope, easy, with just me and my little computer. I have so many solid personal contacts that I could go to each of them right now, make eye contact, firmly shake their hand, and say in a sincere voice, "John/Jennifer, I need $10 from you. Don't ask me why, I just need it. Will you give it to me?" I would get some "no's" of course, but the percentage would be small. The more intimate the contact, the more I'd ask for and vice-versa. Messrs. Jones and Smith from Kroger's might only give me five or ten, but Messrs. Come and Taylor would probably give me $100—or even $500 -$1,000. And you can't believe how much computer software I have filled with people just like them. I get out amongst 'em, ladies and gentlemen. Do you realize how many former students alone would give me $5 - $10. (Don't say it! I already know that there are some who wouldn't give me the time of day. But not too many and I'll cover the "no's" in the next chapter).

C) A MORE REALISTIC EXAMPLE

The first two examples were probably too "far-out" for you—as they are for me—but they are still true. But, just in case you think they are "rubbish," let me give you a true example in order to let you know that I'm not just an "ivory-tower," "pie-in-the-sky" professor with not enough sense to come in out of the rain—a common stereo type of college professors. You are reading this book right now. It is my sincere hope that you feel that it is very practical and worth your time and money. It is further my fervent desire that you think it is GREAT, written very personally, and worth far more than you paid for it. But let's assume for a moment that it's worthless to you or not worth the paper it's written on. Well, I'm going to be pretty "sick" about that—and I'll deeply regret it the rest of my life—but I'll still regret it while I'm walking to the bank.

How can such a confident statement be made before the book is even published? It hasn't even sold one copy yet, has it? Oh, yes it has! My trusty little computer and I got on the phone three weeks before final publishing and PRE-SOLD 2,000 copies of this book to people who didn't know if it was to be any good or not. You see, the Messrs. Jones, Smith, and Fritz from Kroger's all pre-bought one and so did 19 out of every 20 (literally) of my other human relations contacts. I had almost no "no's" and even 95% of those were borderline contacts that I hadn't developed very well. Since I'll make about $2.50 royalties on each book, I've already made $5,000 on this book if not another copy sells.

AND ARE YOU READY FOR THIS? Due to time limitations, I've only scratched the surface of my computer software. I can spend another year or two calling them all just in Ohio alone. Boasting? Well, maybe so, but I'm sharing a very personal experience with you (and I.R.S.) to prove to you that I've done nothing that you also can't do. And maybe this book will "go national" and hit it big. I've certainly read books of this type (self-improvement) that have been top-sellers that are not as good as this one.

SPECIAL NOTE

You might like to know that when you contact people you have known, once in a while (not often) you will find someone who literally ENJOYS saying "no" to you. You can tell that they found some reason for not liking you (all of us "rub" some people the wrong way) and that they delight in rubbing your nose in a "no." Little do they know that I overcame the fear of the word "no" many years go. It is a great "gift" for you to possess also (if you are truly success-oriented) and I'll show you how in the next chapter.

CONCLUSION

The Walkian Formula for Certain Success is continued in the next chapter. In the meantime, begin to practice your eight human relations skills. And make no mistake, they can be both practiced and developed. They are not inborn or inherited. Only lack of positive self-image inhibits their usage. And your tri-lateral programming, "pills", and subsequent weight-loss will soon be taking care of that. Let us march onward!

CHAPTER THIRTEEN

The Success Formula Continues

D) LOW ABASEMENT, HIGH ACHIEVEMENT, LOW INFAVOIDANCE

Over many years of living life and teaching, I have tried to analyze what makes people succeed and what makes them fail. More explicitly, I've attempted to study carefully what has made me succeed (I count many successes) and what has caused me to fail (to list all my failures would indeed be embarrassing). Besides those factors already listed previously, the Terrific Triumverate I'm about to discuss—or the Terrible Triumverate, if they are not followed succinctly—is highly essential. People who are able to work themselves UPWARD on ACHIEVEMENT need scales and DOWNWARD on ABASEMENT need and INFAVOIDANCE need scales almost always succeed greatly. Those individuals who stay low on achievement scales and/or high on abasement and infavoidance scales seldom experience anything but "loserism." Let's examine all three explicitly and carefully, because they are significant keys in unlocking your full potentials and moving you toward a position of self-actualization.

ABASEMENT

If someone says to you that "You're not attractive" or "You're not intelligent" or "You're not a good parent" or "You should feel guilty or ashamed," etc., they are debasing you. On the other hand, if you say to yourself "I am not attractive" or "I'm not very intelligent" or "I'm not a good parent" or "I feel guilty or ashamed," you are ABASING yourself. Bottom line: Abasement is to punish oneself; to feel sorry for self; to self-destruct in one of the hundreds of ways we self-destruct; or to give into fate. It is to get down on yourself or to "cry in your beer." It is to wallow in self-pity. Even more basic, it is to feel as though the universe, life, and daily living situations have control over you rather than you having control over most of them. By nature, we all abase ourselves to some extent. Anytime you know an action you take is destructive to you in anyway, yet you continue to participate in that activity, then you are too high on abasement scales for your own well-being (yes, obsessive-compulsive eating is one of those activities). Sigmund Freud detailed to us almost a century ago the nature of—and strength of—the death instinct in all of us. Abasement is the death instinct personified—either on a mild basis ("rainy day feelings") or a severe basis (suicide). But many persons slowly and surely commit suicide each day. They haven't the courage to shoot themselves or jump off a bridge—so they consciously or unconsciously destroy their own being. In psychological terms, they have high abasement needs. But most all of us are higher than we should be, or need be, on abasement scales. And ANY time we spend in abasement activities is not only self-defeating, but wasted time. It serves absolutely no purpose—plus it cripples us emotionally and hinders our growth and development. Success-type people are either, by nature, low abasement persons or people who are able to recognize their abasement and work themselves cognitively (knowingly) DOWN on the scale. I have gone through extended periods of life in which I was a strong "nine" on abasement scales. Those were largely failure times. Now I am at most a "three" and striving quickly to reach "two," "one," and "zero" (though impossible). However, I now spend very little time punishing myself. You should not either. Part of the NEW YOU should be to steadily move yourself DOWN on abasement scales. It's the only way to a reasonably successful, contented, relaxing life.

Harken back to my Hustler Parable in an earlier chapter. George C. Scott readily recognized that Fast Eddie (Paul Newman) was a person with high abasement needs and, therefore, was fairly certain (certain enough to wager a large amount of money) that Minnesota Fats would eventually do him in.

HIGH ACHIEVEMENT

Murray, one of our most noted psychologists and educators, many years ago detailed the 20 basic psychological needs that all of us manifest. In my opinion, Murray's needs are still the best description of human personality available today. He has stood the test of time—the true barometer of greatness. For what it's worth, no psychologist has even come close to passing the test of time as has Sigmund Freud. To this day, though many do not admit it, almost EVERY psychologist—in one way or another—builds off of and/or borrows and steals from "SIGGY-BABY." Those same psychologists often damn him and will not admit one FACT: Almost without exception, EVERY ONE of Freud's major theories have now either been proven true or are well-documented and well-accepted in our field. And I have no doubts that, as soon as the field of pupillametrics is more perfected, even Freud's most controversial areas of oedipus complex, electra complex, penis envy, castration complex, feces withholding, etc. will be proved beyond a shadow of a doubt. For example, I would bet my life that through pure instinct, every four-year-old girl's (except possibly those with hormonal imbalances which makes them more "male" than "female") eye pupils will dilate (proving pleasurable experience) when shown an erect penis—either live or by picture—thus proving Freud's "penis envy" concept. I'll further wager that every four-year-old boy's (except possibly those with hormonal imbalance which makes them more "female" than "male") eye pupils will contract (showing threat) when a man's hand moves near to his genitals—thus proving the castration complex.

Enough of the commercial for Freud, though I remind you that obsessive-compulsive eating is quite Freudian. In fact, I think you'll find that he coined the term obsessive-compulsive. Let's get back to Murray and his needs. Just as Murray outlined the need of abasement, so also did he well-delineate achievement. It is as follows:

ACHIEVEMENT DEFINED

TO ACCOMPLISH SOMETHING DIFFICULT. TO MASTER, MANIPULATE OR ORGANIZE PHYSICAL OBJECTS, HUMAN BE-INGS OR IDEAS. TO DO THIS AS RAPIDLY AND AS IN-DEPENDENTLY AS POSSIBLE. TO OVERCOME OBSTACLES AND ATTAIN A HIGH STANDARD. TO EXCEL ONESELF. TO RIVAL AND SURPASS OTHERS. TO INCREASE SELF-REGARD BY THE SUCCESSFUL EXERCISE OF TALENT.

I'm sure you know someone who possesses extremely high achievement needs. Actually, the need to achieve can be too high if it's for the wrong reasons. Yet, it can't possibly be too high if it's for the right reasons. Permit me to elaborate. To achieve is to have the need to accomplish something difficult; to rival and surpass others; and to do so as rapidly and as independently as possible. We can all recount many noted people—including entertainers, businessmen, doctors, athletes, actors and actresses, authors, etc.—who have been DRIVEN to achieve highly, and have done so, yet are obviously highly unhappy and therefore self-destruct (ABASEMENT). The world is full of the Elvises'; the Judy Garlands'; the Marilyn Monroes', etc.—persons who have seemingly conquered the world, yet live lives of quiet despondence. Why? It is my contention that they achieved highly for the wrong reasons—either a) due to the fear of intimidation of a significant person(s) in their early life (usually parents or siblings—but not always) or b) the unconscious need to prove themselves to a significant person who has deprived them in some manner. To cite just one quick example: It is my contention that the reason there is such a significant percentage of highly successful—yet unhappy—doctors is because far too many go into medicine for the wrong reasons. That is, they succumb to parental pressure (intimidation), for money, power, prestige, and status. Achievement for the sake of pleasing others by meeting their expectations and standards is almost always hollow and meaningless. That appears to me to be a universal truth. Yet, one can be a "ten" on achievement scales with no difficulty if it is for the right reasons. That is, a wholesome desire to simply be the best you can be within the time span you are allotted on this earth. When you come to the realization that the true meaning to life is to grow; develop; become more fully human; create and reach potentials for yourself and by YOUR standards—then, and only then, will you gain true satisfaction from your achievements—at least in a beneficial way. I know of what I speak here.

I achieved much from the time I was 16 until I was 36. But I achieved for the wrong reasons—responsibility to family—and I spent those 20 prime years of my life largely in quiet desperation or miserably unhappy. On the surface I had it all: A nice wife; wonderful children; money; academic degrees; administrative teaching and coaching success; honors of all types; public speaking requests galore; etc. Yet I was "hurting" and unfulfilled, a driven man wildly bent on living up to others' expectations; an out of control "whirling dirvish" trying always to prove myself. Not only did I not "stop to smell the roses," I thought it was a dumb idea. Aw, but now? I'm still very high on achievement needs, but whatever I accomplish—big or small—is done for the right reasons. I no longer live my life by parental, familial, societal, ministerial, journalistic, academic or ritualistic standards. I live by the principles of SELF-CONCEPT and SELF-GROWTH. I urge you to do it, also. It's the ONLY way to go if life is to be meaningful in a modern, high-tech world. "Sure it's a tough ole world, but let's get on with it."

TIME OUT FOR PARENTS!

I have placed a great deal of emphasis already in this book upon the importance of early learning, early teaching, and early parental environment and the significant role they play on an individual's life-long development. Almost any psychiatrist, therapeutic psychologist, or teacher of psychology would, by necessity have to agree with me. Freud placed great emphasis upon same. So even did the Bible with the classic quote, "Bring up a child in the way he should go and he'll never part from it."

Therefore, I have found that many people (including a large number of my students) like to use these early environmental experiences (especially traumatic ones) as cop-outs on life. "The reason I'm so messed up is because of my parents" or "It's your fault mom and/or dad that I have all the hang-ups I have."

Interestingly, however, though you may well be absolutely correct, you still CANNOT BLAME YOUR PARENTS FOR YOUR PERSONALITY DEFECTS! Why not, you say? If it's basically their fault, then why can't I blame them, by golly? Well, you see, if you are correct, then why do you give your parents such a rough, conflicting time, but often get along so well with grandma and grandpa? If I were your father or mother, I would say to you, "If you are right, my son, that the way I raised you has made you the weirdo you are, then I'm the neurotic mess I am because of your grandparents. Don't blame me. Go lay your troubles on them."

And, of course, if I were your grandfather, when you approached me with your kinkiness, I'd tell you to go visit your great-grandpa up on Boot Hill.

The point here is that you can blame no one—EVEN IF IT IS THEIR FAULT! You can only gain insight into your own conduct and go about changing it by the principles outlined in this book. Don't rationalize—just actualize!

LOW INFAVOIDANCE

Aha! Here is the real key to my entire success formula. I love to discuss it in my class, in my speeches, and with you. Murray's actual definition of infavoidance is as follows:

TO AVOID HUMILIATION. TO QUIT EMBARRASSING SITUATIONS OR TO AVOID CONDITIONS WHICH MAY LEAD TO BELITTLEMENT: THE SCORN, DERISION, OR THE INDIFFERENCE OF OTHERS. TO REFRAIN FROM ACTION BECAUSE OF THE FEAR OF FAILURE.

Put in simple terms, infavoidance is our grave fear of the word "no" and our fear of failure. And all of us are higher than we should be in infavoidance! Because we are so ego-centric—that is, focused in so strongly on our own being, identity, and security—we become overly anxious about being embarrassed; having people laugh at us; failing; being turned down; etc. Therefore, as Murray states, WE REFRAIN FROM ACTION BECAUSE OF A FEAR OF FAILURE. I would easily be a multi-millionaire right now if it weren't for my being too high on the scale of infavoidance. Probably the same is true of you. In a free enterprise society, MAKING MONEY IS SO EASY. It doesn't even take much intelligence. It is INFAVOIDANCE which hinders and detours your success—not intelligence. Let me cite a few quick examples: 1) Most of you will say that you now wish you could play a musical instrument. What kept you from learning? Or keeps you from learning now? Infavoidance! 2) Most of us proclaim that we would have liked to be famous entertainers, politicians, actors, etc. What prevented us from so doing? Pure infavoidance. You don't think Ernest Borgnine, Barbara Stanwick, Roy Rogers, Ronald Reagan, etc. possess any more abilities or good looks than most of you, do you? Absolutely not! They simply were low enough on infavoidance scales so as not to be afraid to give it a try. They weren't afraid of being embarrassed or the word "no." 3) There are so many good singers, dancers, model prospects, etc. in this country who'll never perform because "I can't perform very well—I'll bet people would laugh." A combination of abasement and infavoidance. 4) There are thousands (probably millions) of Americans right now who would like to start their own business. Why don't they? They're afraid they would fail and they, therefore, quake at the risk. Progress always involves risk. You can't steal second and keep on foot on first!

When discussing infavoidance I always like to use one of my favorite persons as an example—the incomparable Willie Nelson. He truly is an example of low infavoidance. The "Nashville Mafia"—the powers-that-be who controlled country music for years—laughed at Willie, ignored him, and for the most part excluded him. They told him he couldn't sing and, by classic standards, he can't. Terrible nasal quality. They told him he couldn't play the guitar very well. In truth there are probably thousands of musicians who CAN play it as well. They told him his songs were no good, and that he'd never be a successful songwriter. They in essence told him to go back to Texas and sell shoes. They later told him his hair was too long, his beard too scraggly, and his face too leathery to be a music star and movie star. Most of us would have been back in our hometowns selling shoes years ago, but not Willie. Willie had the great gift of low-infavoidance. Willie possessed perserverance—the by-word of low infavoidance and the password to success. Willie would not, in street terms, take "no" for an answer. Ole Willie was as unsinkable as Molly Brown. He had learned that the "chase" is more important that the "catch," anyway (see last chapter).

And you know the results, do you not? Willie is now the king! Not even

Kenny Rogers or Dolly "Feet-in-the-Shade" Parton can compare. His nasal voice IS a classic. His guitar playing is homey and superb. He takes an audience of 20,000 and makes each member feel as though he's playing in his backyard for a family picnic. His songs continually hit the top. And listen to this: Most women actually saw him as a sex symbol in "Honeysuckle Rose" due to his gentleness, his sincerity, his tender eyes, and his natural charisma. At his concerts, he will stay as long as a significant part of the audience wishes to listen. But we never would have known the joys of Willie Nelson had he not had LOW INFAVOIDANCE NEEDS. Like us, he would have pulled up his stakes, hung his head in shame, and crawled home long ago. Infavoidance is the greatest crippler of success known of man! "If you have a FEAR of losing, you'll never be a winner" . . . (Dizzy Dean).

THE GIRL SCOUT PARABLE

I teach often by parable and concept. It is one of my major trademarks as a teacher—and I love teaching. Following is my favorite infavoidance parable. As with any parable, apply it to any and every situation you wish. There were once two Girl Scouts—Hortense and Katherine. It was Girl Scout Cookie selling time and the scoutmaster had handed out cookie allotments for sales. Each scout had been informed that whomever sold the most cookies would win an all-expense paid trip to Disneyland.

Hortense, for whatever environmental causes, was a high infavoidance young girl. Katherine, no matter the originating factors, was a low infavoidance young female. Hortense, like all high infavoidance persons, was so insecure (lack of ego strength and identity) that being embarrassed in any way was "crushing" to her. She just could not handle rejection; she simply deplored the indifference of others; humilitation was torture; and the word "no" reduced her to nothingness.

Therefore, Hortense sold her cookies to mom and dad (no "no's" there). She sold a couple of boxes to grandma and grandpa (how could grandparents ever say no?). Her brother and his wife bought a box—though asking them was highly anxiety-producing to her. Fortified with all her "success," Hortense ventured out into the world (ha!). She went next door to Mrs. Jones' house. In a typical high-infavoidance fashion, she timidly knocked on the door. When Mrs. Jones appeared, Hortense dropped her chin and eyes and said softly, "I don't suppose you'd want to buy any Girl Scout Cookies, would you?"

Mrs. Jones, a harsh, bitter "bad milk baby" type of person, retorts coldly, "No Hortense. I do NOT want any Girl Scout Cookies."

That's it. Girl Scout Cookie selling time is over for Hortense. She "crawls" home; withdraws into the TV or bedroom; and turns in her $5.00

and an entire box of unsold cookies to the scoutmaster two weeks later. And, tragically, unless she undergoes major change (possibly reading this book would be a start), her life patterns are already established. High infavoidance will haunt her the remainder of her life. Her success levels—by any definition—do not have a very good prognosis. She's destined to dwell in the shadows of the avenues, forever.

Aw, but let's peer in at Katherine and her Girl Scout Cookie selling approach. Katherine is a very low-infavoidance person who has little fear of rejection due to more than ample identity strength. Naturally, selling to ALL her family is "no sweat!" She'll even find relatives mom and dad might not even know existed. So, it becomes time to explore and exploit the outer universe. No problem! And, just for the sake of making a point, let's say she lives in the same neighborhood as Hortense. So, she first stops by Mrs. Jones' home—ole witch woman herself. As "Crabapple" appears, Katherine begins her confident spiel, "Hi, Mrs. Jones, it's Girl Scout Cookie time again. They're better this year than ever—and we even have three new flavors. How many boxes would you like?"

Mrs. Jones responds indignantly, "Young lady, Hortense has already been here. I told her what I'll tell you. I don't eat cookies and I most certainly don't want to buy any Girl Scout Cookies."

But Katherine is unscathed. "They're especially delicious this year, Mrs. Jones. Maybe your grandchildren or nieces and nephews have a birthday soon. They make very nice gifts!"

Jonesy defiantly reacts. "I told you, Katherine. I do NOT want any cookies."

"Well, thank you anyway," says Katherine softly and politely, "Maybe I'll stop back later if I have any cookies left. Good-bye!"

Katherine then proceeds next door to Mrs. Smith's. Her self-esteem has already overcome Mrs. Jones rudeness. Without realizing it, she has established in her mind that Mrs. Jones' problem is her (Mrs. Jones') own problem and not one personal to her (Katherine). In addition, without realizing it, she has an internalized "gift" that will make her eternally successful.

"Hi, Mrs. Smith! How are you today? It's Girl Scout Cookie time again," she exclaims enthusiastically. "Our cookies are super this year and we have new flavors. How many boxes would you like to buy?"

"Thank you, Katherine, for stopping by," Mrs. Smith says cordially. "But I don't think I'll buy any this year."

"Have you considered buying them as gifts for your family, Mrs. Smith? They DO make nice birthday or holiday gifts."

"No, thank you. I don't think so, Kathi. But I'll give it some thought."

"O. K., Mrs. Smith. I'll stop back if I have any cookies left."

"Fine, Katherine," states Mrs. Smith, certain that she has seen the last of Kathi.

Katherine then simply journies next door to Mr. Spencer's home.

"Good afternoon, Mr. Spencer. It's Girl Scout Cookie time again. They're great this year and we have some super new flavors. How many boxes would you like?"

"Why, Kathi, your timing is perfect. I'm just making coffee and am in the mood to please my sweet tooth. Do you have peanut butter cookies?"

"Oh, yes, Mr. Spencer—and they're very fresh," says Katherine positively.

"I'll take a box. No, make that two because I'm visiting the widow Scott this afternoon and I think I'll take her a box."

Kathi continues, "Mr. Spencer, do you have any family members with special occasions coming up? These make very nice gifts."

Mr. Spencer reflects briefly. "I'm glad you mentioned it, Kathi. My twin grandchildren DO have a birthday in two weeks. You'd better give me two boxes of peanut butter and two of chocolate chip. They like both."

Well, you already know what's going to happen, don't you? Katherine is going to sell a potful of cookies; gain even more self-concept than she now possesses; and spend a week at Disneyland. All just because she is low on infavoidance scales. What a cheap price to pay for high level success. Perseverance has always won out over talent.

However, the parable is not complete yet. One week prior to sales' deadline, Katherine still has a carton of cookies remaining of the 17 cases she has already sold. So she approaches Mrs. Jones' door again. "Hi, Mrs. Jones, how are you today!" she says politely, "I have a few boxes of cookies left and thought you might like some for yourself or as gifts."

"Young lady," Jonesy retorts, "I've already told you that I don't want any cookies."

"Well, thank you anyway, Mrs. Jones, I just thought I'd check. It's nice to see you again."

Katherine then bee-lines it to Mrs. Smith's home. "Hi, Mrs. Smith, I have a few boxes of cookies left and thought you might be interested in some."

"Well, thank you Katherine, I've just been hoping you'd stop back. I forgot that my twin nieces are having a birthday party next week and I don't want their mother baking for all those children at the party. I would like to have 15 boxes if you have that many left."

"Oh yes," says Katherine happily." And I still have a nice selection, too. Thank you very much!"

Now it is one day before sales are over and Kathi still has one box remaining. You guessed it. There she goes to ole' Mrs. Jones House. "Hi, Mrs. Jones, this is my last day and I have one box of cookies left. Would you like it."

"O.K., O.K., Mrs. Jones responds in an exasperated tone, "I'll take them." She either buys them to get rid of the little brat or because she admires Kathi's stick-to-itiveness. Either way, Kathi doesn't care. She only knows that she sold the cookies.

There are many valid and reliable research studies on sales and any quality salesman will tell you that he doesn't even expect to make a sale until the third visit. The Hortense's of this world cannot even comprehend third visits. With the Katherine's, third visits are commonplace.

As mentioned previously, you can aptly apply this parable to ANY situation you wish—from selling encyclopedias to selling oil tankers; from playing country music to becoming a politician; and from acting to selling widgets. THROUGHOUT THE HISTORY OF THE WORLD, NERVE AND PERSEVERANCE HAVE ALWAYS TRIUMPHED OVER TALENT AND LUCK 90% OF THE TIME! Naturally, having all four makes the world your oyster.

So, if you can just work at moving yourself DOWN on abasement and infavoidance scales and UP on achievement scales—combined with hard work, hard play, and human relations skills—there is little you cannot accomplish. But we're not even near complete with the formula as yet. Let's go for it all!

SPECIAL NOTE

I've already related to you that I've had many successes in my life and many more failures. Yet, I've always been a very enterprising person (high achievement)—all of an honest, legitimate nature. I would easily be a multi-millionaire now because of my creative ideas—except for infavoidance. My insecurity and lack of identity strength made me an unhealthy "eight" on in-favoidance scales during the prime years of my life—just as I spent those years grossly overweight. I'll NEVER make those two errors again. DON'T YOU EITHER!

THE STORY
OF THE VIETNAMESE WOMAN

Let me tell you a true story now to sum up my point that money is so easy to make if one A) Has good human relations skills; B) Is high on achievement scales and low on abasement and infavoidance scales, and C) Is creative—which will be discussed in a subsequent chapter.

About six months ago, I was sitting in my office at the college and experienced something unique in my 10 years at Shawnee State. There was a knock at my door and before I could even answer, the door opened and a diminutive, cute, well-dressed Vietnamese woman quietly entered. She held before my eyes two bamboo reed wall mats with Oriental pictures, began nodding her head up and down, and smiling, mumbling in Oriental tones. I could not understand her but realized that she wanted to know if I wanted to purchase one or more of the mats. I inquired as to whether they were hand-painted and she kept nodding and chanting, not really answering my question, but implying that they were. I then asked, "How much?"

That she understood and quickly answered in broken English with Oriental dialect, "Eighta-feefty, eighta-feefty ($8.50).

I said "no, thank you." She nodded most politely, bowed to me quickly, and proceeded down the row of faculty offices, stopping at each door to repeat her sales ritual. Actually, such soliciting is unlawful on state property but who is going to call the police on such a delightful little lady?

A few minutes later, I went to the men's room and noticed that she was selling a couple of wall mats to one of our faculty members. In the next three minutes, she sold five more. The next day I learned that she had gone into our library and all of our college buildings. I, personally, could account for 17 mats that she had sold on her "whirlwind" journey of our campus. Rest assured, there were more.

About an hour later, my day was over and I ventured to the nearby Ramada Inn Lounge for a little R. and R. I was sitting in the lounge with a friend, John, discussing the events of the day and solving the problems of the world. In came "Vera Vietnam" and began doing her thing. She didn't recognize me and humbly approached John and me with her now familiar (but not to John) pitch. John perused the mats and stated, "Tomorrow is my wife's birthday and I think she'd like those. Are they hand-painted?"

Vera's head just kept bobbing as if on a spring and John soon bought one for "eighta feefty." After the purchase, Vera reached into a small bag and held out an empty box to John—obviously so that he would effectively wrap his gift. I noted the "Made in Taiwan" on the box and John and I both realized (and discussed) that the mat probably cost her at most 50 cents—and probably even less. "Oh, well, it still looks nice and will make Brenda a nice gift," John rationalized.

I was now becoming even more intrigued by "Vera," especially since she sold five more mats in the lounge—and soliciting there is also against the law. But would you arrest "Vera?" Then you probably beat children, throw rocks at dogs, and tie your grandmother's panties in knots, don't you?

So when "Vera" made her hasty exit, I conveniently went to the men's room again. Out in the lobby, Viet Vera had drawn a crowd of railroad workers staying at the motel, and she sold six more mats in a five minute span. It's safe to say she'd just profited $48.00 from those railroaders. I was in awe!

Vera was cleaned out. She bowed politely and departed out the back lobby door. I was now magnetized and had to follow—at a distance, of course. She went through the parking lot and behind the motel. I soon stealthily peered around the corner of the building and saw just about what I'd expected to see.

Parked along the curb was a slickly-dressed, slick-haired caucasian man in a new, white El Dorado Cadillac. The classy car was packed to capacity with cardboard cartons (wonder what was in them?) and, as "Vera" approached, he got out of the car and opened the trunk—filled with similar cartons. He handed the appealing woman another bagful of reed wall mats and away she went. You can imagine my thoughts at that moment.

That evening, I purposely made the rounds of Portsmouth's motels and soon found the easily-discernible El Dorado at the Holiday Inn and found the "pimp" and his woman eating giant steaks in the motel restaurant. I later learned that they also spent the next day "pillaging" the depressed city at the mouth of the port of the Ohio and Scioto Rivers. She "worked" the banks, the public library, the streets, and the restaurants.

Conservatively, I figure that Mr. El Dorado and Vera Vietnam left our fair city with $2,000 in clear profit in two days and then moved on to the next green pastures. Please keep in mind that A) Portsmouth is basically a down-on-its-luck city and B) That Internal Revenue would have difficulty keeping tabs on this couple. If I were Mr. Caucasian, I would treat "Meal Ticket Vera" with great respect and dignity. For as long as she remains in good health—and the Taiwanese keep producing bamboo reed wall mats with cheap labor—Mr. "Slicko" is going to make profits by the potful. And you think money isn't easy to make? Shows what you know!

E) WHOLESOME SELF-CONCEPT INCLUDING PRIDE IN PERSONAL APPEARANCE AND GROOMING

This entire book is based on self-concept psychology and the principles for achieving it. But I've found that rarely do you meet someone who TRULY has a good self-image who does not take pride in his/her personal appearance, dress, and grooming. There is no doubt that one dresses and grooms for success. There is just too much research to prove that clothes and grooming do NON-VERBALLY communicate our intentions and dictate how well—or how poorly—we reach our goals. If you do not realize this truism, you are quite foolish! Nothing succeeds like success! And clothes and grooming DO make the man—and woman!

YOUR BODY SCENT

The most intimate thing we humans do is to participate in sexual intercourse. BUT, the most personal thing we have is the scent (or odor) of our bodies. In this day and age, there is ABSOLUTELY NO EXCUSE for any person not smelling nicely except during physical exercise or exertion. Even as a college professor, I never cease to be amazed how many students give off either a highly negative body odor or some strong cologne-type scent that overwhelms those around them. At least three or four times annually, other students approach me and inform me that they cannot even tolerate to sit in the vicinity of Sammy Sweat or Sally Sour. A quick bit of "experiential research" shows me that they're correct. Sally and Sammy need to least invent a new deodorant called "Disperse" (it doesn't kill the smell, but spreads it out so you can't tell who it's coming from. Ha!).

Seriously, you should continually strive to give off a pleasant scent and continually search for the deodorants, colognes, powders, and aftershaves which are "you"—that is, those chemicals which best combine with your body chemistry to create a pleasant smell. This body chemistry is important and must not be overlooked or underestimated. For example, have you ever smelled the older woman who over-uses lilac and the lilac combined with her aging body chemistry creates an overpowering aroma somewhere between toilet water and death?

You need to experiment and "conduct research" on your body smell. Surprisingly, it is not difficult to do. You see, as stated previously, seldom will anyone tell you that you smell badly and seldom will anyone tell you that you smell nicely unless they really mean it. Furthermore, if you DO really smell good, a significant number of people will comment on it. So, experiment and research until you get "quite a few" people commenting on your odiferous nature over a period of a week. THEN YOU HAVE FOUND THE SCENT—at least for the time being!

Let me relate an interesting personal experience: The first scent I used as a young boy/man when I first started shaving was Mennen's Skin Bracer (aftershave). Since that time I have probably tried almost every scent on the market for extended periods of time. But now, as a 46-year-old man, I get the most compliments from those around me when I wear Mennen's Aftershave. And, just for the record, I also use Right Guard anti-perspirant—the best sweat gland retarder I've found; Johnson's Baby Powder on my body—the greatest scent ever invented, in my opinion; and Johnson's Baby Shampoo on my hair. That's it!

PERSONAL GROOMING

Angee Whitt, whom I acknowledged in the beginning of this book—and have referred to frequently since—has taught me much the past few years about personal grooming. Because of her contributions, she must be considered a collaborating author of this book. She is an R.N. and a model and she possesses much knowledge about grooming, dress, make-up (women), etc. far beyond her years—for both men and women. Before I met Angee, I was clean, make no mistake about that. But I was not well-groomed or well-dressed—and did not, quite frankly, even know what they meant. Let me give some typical examples:

A) HAIR

I simply got my hair cut when I thought I needed it. And it was just that—a hair cut. I considered styling something that only actors and male homosexuals did. "Styling," it seemed to me, was waviness or curliness, or something else negative. Angee taught me that styling your hair is nothing of the sort—that it's just a stylish cut which compliments your head, face, ear structure, etc.

My hair is very thin on top. I'm not happy about it, but I'm not vain and sensitive, either. However, I had frustratedly "given up" and didn't care anymore. Angee taught me how to sweep my hair back on the sides, style the sides and back, and look as nice as it is possible to look with my obvious limitations. AND THIS IS THE POINT OF ALL GROOMING AND DRESS—TO LOOK AS NICE AS POSSIBLE, NOT VANITY! I could not believe the difference she created in my appearance with simple architectural changes in my hair.

B) ALL OTHER BODY HAIR

We established long ago the Freudian significance of hair on a man. The manner in which he handles ALL his hair is culturally highly important—both to the men and women around him. The same is true regarding the way women handle ALL their hair. Quite honestly, I'd never given much thought to all this. Just let it go—and grow—naturally.

For example, I never (or seldom) trimmed my now thick and bushy eyebrows. I never even gave it much thought. Now I do! I only trimmed the hair from my nose periodically. Yuk! Not true now. (Am I ringing some bells?) I had superficial hair growing all over my ears and back and neck. Now it is either removed (ears) or kept trimmed (back and neck).

I wore a beard in winter, mustache in fall and spring, and went clean-shaven in summer. In none of those seasons was any of my facial hair well-kept or fastidiously shaven. Not so now!

Finally, sometimes I would show my hairy chest ostentatiously, sometimes not at all. But there was no organization or purpose to either. Not so now! I pick my spots and my occasions to "flash" or "not to flash" quite carefully—depending on the situation and what I wish to accomplish. There is much research to show that men can "make or break" themselves by the manner of and strategy with which they utilize all body hair.

C) OTHER BODY FEATURES

Fingernails, toenails, body tone, body building, etc. All these things are important to a person who is wanting to develop himself/herself to the fullest in an allotted period on this earth. So is posture, carriage, make-up (women), etc. You don't need to be neurotic about all this—just reasonably conscientious. Do not overlook the proper care and use of these features!

D) CLOTHES AND DRESSING IN THEM

If you are to be successful, you must first look and smell successful. You may realize that there has been a best seller book on the market the past decade on successful dressing. I highly recommend the reading of that book. It is very, very good. My only reservation about it is its conservatism (probably necessary) and the fact that it has become the "Wall Street Bible" and thus created a mass conformity, Madison Avenue robot which scares the heck out of me. A prime example: In the book it tells how the beige raincoat is a symbol of upper middle class and the black raincoat is a symbol of lower middle class. The author presents research to back his claim. He's no doubt correct. Trouble is, anyone who IS ANYONE has now read his book. Therefore, this past December, when I visited my daughter in Philadelphia—and it was raining—all of downtown Philly was a sea of clones wearing beige raincoats. How boring and 1984-ish. He also shows how dark suits and long sleeve, white dress shirts bring respect and power in the corporate world. You don't suppose his brother is in the dark suit and long sleeve dress shirt business, do you? If not, he darn well should be! Nevertheless, the book is must reading as far as I'm concerned. But I wish to add some of my own thoughts (and Angee's) also.

DRESSING
THE MAN FOR ACHIEVEMENT

First of all, seldom do you meet a successful person who does not have shoes shined or his clothes neatly pressed. Now you can relate to me, I'm sure, all kinds of exceptions. But they are still EXCEPTIONS, NOT RULES. Keep your shoes shined and your clothes pressed. If in doubt as to whether you'll be showing your underwear on a given day, press them, (that's a joke, son, but a good cardinal rule to follow).

Secondly, match colors and lines carefully—always! Not only do women notice it astutely, but I'm convinced that males respect other males who do so—even if unconsciously. Color-coding is invaluable. All the way from glasses to the tie to sox (and underwear—if the day's activities might warrant).

Thirdly, you do not have to spend big amounts of money to have a wardrobe of variety and excellence. If you have ample resources—fine! But, if you do not, using limited monies as an excuse for poor dress is flat-out a cop-out. There are great bargains to be had everywhere and mix-n-match permits you to have only seven or eight complete outfits and appear to wear a different outfit EVERY DAY OF THE YEAR! Even every day for five years in the case of women! It's pure mathematics. The key is to seldom (or never) buy an outfit that isn't carefully selected to match with most of the other garb you already have in your closet. Soon you build a wardrobe similar to Wendy's Hamburgers—you can fix them 256 ways. Though this is even easier for a woman (due to hats, headbands, earrings, and high heels), it can still be accomplished quite readily by men. And if you really have your head together, both women and men can purchase expensive, practically-new outfits at yard sales for $2.00.

Fourthly, you must make a psychological decision each day—or evening—whether it is to your benefit to dress for visibility, non-visibility, flamboyance, conservatism, etc. Your ability to do this properly is crucial. Let me give you some quick hints: A) If in doubt in an important situation, dress more conservative, B) but don't be afraid to be different—so long as you're not outlandish. People remember different! C) You are always a threat or a "show" when you over-dress. D) Develop a "Trademark"—a type of general dress that you become known for MOST (not all) of the time—but it must be something that is "you." Mine happens to be suspenders, though they're not really in style right now. E) And that reminds me, don't let "what's in style" bother you so long as MOST people like you in it and have come to accept you in that garb. F) Do not be threatened to ask others' opinion of how you look. The best approach here is to take pictures and have them submitted (through friends) to people who do not even know you and ask them to evaluate your appearance and ways to improve it. (Friends have so many built in bias' and halo's that they'll either tell you you look super when you don't or "smart-assedly" recommend a team of plastic surgeons and Paris designers).

I am convinced that there is no such thing as a plain or homely person. Any person who takes pride in their personal body and appearance and who continually searches for better methods to improve dress and grooming can be at least REASONABLY attractive—if not better. Let me relate two classic examples of people whom I observed first-hand change from rather "plain" images (at best) to most attractive (even handsome) images. Both are men and both were clients of mine who had lost substantial weight with my program and were then motivited to be "better looking." We'll call them Tom Cellars and Buck Crain (not their real names).

TOM CELLARS

I discussed Tom earlier but now will tell you about his experiences with clothes and grooming. Tom was a balding man with very oily hair, horn-rimmed glasses, and very dated clothes' styles. I asked his permission to let Angee make some recommendations and "work on him." He readily agreed. He had gone from 260 lbs. to 180 lbs. and had practiced in a Nautilus program which had him toned nicely. But still he had a plain look—even a "seedy" look. Tom was a 5'8", 30-year-old bachelor who women simply avoided.

The changes Angee recommended were so simple and basic—yet so insightful as to be almost genius. Though they would appear to be "right in front of your eyes," Tom could not see them. Frankly, even though I have now become quite conscious of both my appearance and others' appearances, I could not have seen or done what Angee did. She started right at the top and worked down. I was not permitted to be present as Angee wanted a confidential one-to-one relationship with Tom (and I think she also wanted to surprise me since this was our first joint project).

First, she styled Tom's hair and showed him how to shampoo it properly for the "dry look." She slightly swept back his hair on the sides in a neat, stylish, and distinguished look. She instructed him on the art of blow drying and hair spraying so that his thinning hair was not even noticeable. Finally—head-hair wise—she shortened his long, mutton-chop sideburns to normal length and trimmed his over-the-lip, Fu Manchu mustache to a Burt Reynolds' mustache look. Tom's sideburns and mustache had not only given him an unkempt (even dirty) look but accented his short stature and heavy face and jaw line. She also precisely trimmed his bushy eyebrows.

Secondly, she removed his horn-rimmed glasses and fitted him with a very modern-style pair (rims only until he could see his optometrist) that "pulled together" his face—namely, his high forehead and heavy longer face. The selection of glasses—or use of contacts—is SO important in improvement, or impoverishment, of personal appearance. It is astounding the changes you can render with them.

Thirdly, she started to work on clothes' style. Since Tom was almost identical in size to me (except I'm three or four inches taller), she used my wardrobe—much of which she had originally selected—with which to fit Tom. They experimented and made notes regarding dress recommendations for almost two hours. Tom was an avid student and later admitted he had known little about clothes, though he was thirty years old. This is true of most men. And unfortunately, they are usually dressed by women who also know little about dressing men. I'm also completely convinced that most women unconsciously dress their man so that he is unattractive to other women and therefore protect their "property and territory." No one can ever convince me that this isn't true of 90% of women. Furthermore, women do not generally know how to dress men for success in the business world which is mainly controlled by other men (neither do most clerks in mens' stores). In short, few women know diddly-squat about mens' dress. They only know what they like on a man—and don't even usually dress THEIR man in that in fear that other women will try to capture him. Only secure women are the exception to this. Now, before anyone cries "sexist" the exact same is true of men regarding womens' clothes. Only very secure men dress their women (or permit them to garb themselves) so as to be attractive to other men. And few men know absolutely anything about womens' styles in the business or social world. They only know about dressing for the world of sex.

But back to Angee and Tom—and clothes styles. Tom, even though having a college education, had drifted from one state agency job to another and was currently unemployed. No question that lack of self-concept and the accompanying weight problem were major causes of his occupational and professional woes. However, his mode of dress was most certainly a causal factor, also. Tom broke most any and every rule in the book—stripes with plaids; horizontal stripes to accent his shortness and fatness; no color coding; etc. You name it, he botched it. Like most men—even educated, intelligent ones—his knowledge of clothes styles was sadly lacking.

My program had already taken giant strides on the self-concept/weight syndrome. Now it was Angee's turn. She worked with Tom regarding the difference in approach to dressing for work, social life, sportswear, and "sex life." And there ARE major differences. She emphasized finding clothes that are "you." She impressed on Tom the importance of colors and matching lines. Let me briefly outline what she recommended for the 5'8", 180 lb. Tom in terms of clothes. In so doing, you'll see much of her philosophy in mens' dress—most of which I share with her.

She knew that Tom had an interest in the business world. She therefore suggested conservative simplicity in the form of dark, solid color suits; white, long sleeve shirts or white with small vertical pin stripes; and basically solid color ties with modest design in either striping or very small polka dots. Angee believes that not only do dark colors portray power and authority—thereby commanding more respect (proven in many studies), but that dark colors make one look more slender and taller.

She also put major emphasis upon Tom always wearing high heel boots or shoes—not elevator types, but definite high heel. Not only do they legitimately make you taller but they, by structure, usually make you carry yourself in a more positive upright manner when you stand or walk—forcing upper body back a little and stomach in, chest out. The shoulders, back, and buttocks simply manifest themselves—all else being equal—in a more confident manner.

In sports' wear and casual dress, she also recommended solid, dark colors, especially in shirts—and shirts should almost always be darker than slacks. An exception would be the obvious error in wearing dark blue, brown or black on an extremely hot day in the sun due to heat absorption. And, as in all clothes (except some night life attire), the fit is highly important—nothing too loose and baggy, nothing too tight and "flaunty." Also, with short and stocky persons, the cardinal rule of all lines being vertical rather than horizontal is to be followed.

Finally, Angee worked with Tom on "night life" attire, and it was in this garb that I first saw him on his "coming out" night. Angee is a great believer in long sleeve, very large collar, tapered, Spanish-style shirts in which the front is open to clearly show the hair on the chest—but not TOO open and not down to the stomach area. This particular evening, Tom's shirt was pure black. His slacks were also black and fairly tight through his hips and butt—without being obscene—and they were stylish.

He also had on high-heel, black boots. So you must be thinking right now that he looked like a bullfighter at a funeral, right? Wrong! Wait until you hear the rest. First of all, he was wearing a pair of gold rim, high-style glasses. Secondly, he had on a beautiful, choker-style gold chain necklace. His sleeves were turned up one time only, exposing a gold identification bracelet and he had on a gold ring. But now for Angee's genius. She had selected a beautiful pair of thin band, white SUSPENDERS with gold clips and gold adjusters. They were "TOM." They not only made him look taller, but they gave the outfit the color it needed and gave Tom a confident—even mildly cocky, arrogant and aloof look which most women either consciously or unconsciously like in men. (There are studies to prove that this is true with a high percentage of women).

I was sitting in the Ramada Inn in Portsmouth (Portsmouth's best night spot) when Tom walked in. So help me, I did not recognize him with his new hairstyle and everything else just described. I can honestly tell you my first reaction was one of high envy of that "stranger's" outfit as he entered the lounge.

Angee knew I was there and had purposely not entered with Tom. Only when she appeared 30 seconds later did I realize Tom's identity and I was flabbergasted. Sure, I've learned that "clothes make the man," but even I couldn't believe this one. TRULY, FROGS CAN BE TURNED INTO HANDSOME PRINCES! But far more important was Tom's obvious complete change of EVERYTHING—confidence, carriage, and over-all aura—and his words to me as we sat together.

"Jerry," he said, "I cannot believe this! It's as though I'm a new person, and a different man. When I looked in a full-length mirror when Angee finished, my mind was flooded with wonderful thoughts. Thoughts like: Is this me? So help me, even thoughts like: Am I really this good looking? And, why, I look like someone on TV or in the movies."

"And he cried," Angee said softly.

"Yes, I did, Jerry. I cried from happiness; and I cried because I'm 30 years old and didn't learn all this sooner; and I cried because I'm so grateful to both of you. I will always be in your debt."

To finish this entire story rapidly, today Tom is the director of personnel of a medium size manufacturing company. He is married to a wonderful woman and has two great children. He is an impeccably dressed and groomed man. And, as mentioned previously, every Christmas he sends us very expensive gifts which we can't return in kind. But it's the letter which always accompanies those gifts which is most cherished by us, anyway. You see, he thinks we're the greatest thing since indoor plumbing—and that's enough for us.

BUCK CRAIN

Buck is another example of the quality of my program and the ingenius work of Angee with mens' styles. Buck was similar to Tom in a few ways, yet most different in many others. He was a 35-year-old foodaholic. Yet, like a few fortunate obsessive-compulsive eaters, most of his food did not turn to fat. Therefore, he had kind of a weird look in which he didn't possess to much fat except for a very large stomach—a so-called "pot belly" or "beer belly."

Like Tom, Buck was short (5'8") but unlike Tom he had a beautiful head of sandy hair and great facial features (though somewhat camouflaged by his pudginess). Stated simply, it was obvious that Buck would be a very good looking man IF he lost his 30 lb. gut, toned his body, and learned to groom and dress even close to properly. But groom and dress he knew little or nothing about. For example, when we first met him, his idea of a sexy outfit in which to go out "woman-hunting" was a large flowered shirt with plaid pants and penny loafers. I'm dead serious—and believe me those duds were not "HIM!" Buck had heard of my program and reputation and approached me one day seeking help—though I had actually known him for quite a few years. I readily accepted, even though I had a long waiting list. To be honest, the reason is that I like to work with women and men whom it is evident that they have excellent natural attractiveness because 1) it's such a waste of natural beauty to see it covered with fat; 2) they are even more appreciative of the results; and 3) it's just plain easier.

I also told Buck up-front about my partnership with Angee and that I'd like him to hear her out on her recommendations. "No problem," he said, "I want to go all the way. I've seen what it's done for you and your life. You were a sorry-looking character ten years ago." He was feigning humor, but he knew and I knew that he was serious—and correct.

So Buck and I began the entire program detailed in the first half of this book. Like most of my clients, he thought it silly and childish "pretending" at first. But after six weeks, when his "mysterious" thinking and actions began, he became excited. He became almost a complete vegetarian and settled on Nautilus and golf as his regular exercise program. Later, he also "mysteriously" found himself doing the rigorous 20 minute TV exercise program with those beautiful women EVERY morning. He couldn't believe he was doing it (neither could I).

Again, being fortunate not to have a body make-up (metabolism? chemistry?) like most foodaholics, Buck became a slender well-toned man within six months. While most of us do not—and probably should not—lose weight that quickly, please keep in mind that even Buck would have soon gained it back were it not due to the psychological changes in approach to eating that my program elicits—THE ONLY WAY!

So now it was time for Buck to work with Angee and "clean up his act." He met with her for a full two weeks on a one-hour per day basis. In this case, sometimes I was there, sometimes not.

Since his hair was so naturally thick and beautiful (I hate Buck!), Angee really only had to show him how to shampoo and comb it, which she did. But one night she had what turned out to be an idea of brilliance and asked Buck to try it. He had already been so impressed with her many insights that he readily agreed. So, much to my shock, she gave Buck a curly-perm! Yes, an Afro or Gorgeous George-look with Buck's sandy/blonde hair. I broke up laughing at the thought of it because I've never cared for that look on men, anyway. Well, you guessed it, it was "Buck." It looked super and made him look two inches taller. He loved it. And combined with higher heel shoes and vertical lines and stripes, and with his new slenderness, he went from 5'8" to 6'0" overnight. I swear it was like an optical illusion.

Then Angee made another unexpected move. Whereas she thinks most men look nice in glasses IF they're selected carefully, she believed that Buck's naturally great facial bone structure would look better without glasses and suggested contact lenses. He tried them and found her to be correct once again. Together with many of the clothes styles already discussed with Tom (and jewelry—but no suspenders), many of Buck's own acquaintances had difficulty recognizing him. And the women fell all over themselves getting at him. That had not been the case previously. We would take him "partying" with us to Columbus and Cincinnati and he thought he'd died and gone to heaven by the way women would "make themselves available" to him. Another satisfied customer? You bet! He thanks me often—but he flat-out WORSHIPS Angee!

JOIE KOCH

I must relate one more example to you in order to present my (and Angee's) beliefs about women and their dress and grooming. I actually get far more women clients than men (10 to 1) and could cite many cases. But one, in particular, is my favorite over the years. Her name is Joie Koch (prounced Cook) and we are very close friends to this day. You'll see why, I think.

As I sometimes do, I approached Joie as opposed to her coming to me. I do this only when I see a woman who is obviously very beautiful, but also obviously grossly overweight and a foodaholic. And, also, when it at least appears obvious that her fatness is making her unhappy and keeping her from fulfilling her creativity, potential, and human-ness. It wasn't too difficult to see that all this applied to Joie and I asked her to my office. She knew me only as her teacher and I her only as a student. She had no previous knowledge of my program or even my concern with obsessive-compulsive eating and self-concept psychology.

As sincerely and genuinely as possible, I told her my opinions of her beauty; her wasting of that beauty; her foodaholism problem; and the many ways I felt it was debilitating her life. I asked her if she thought I was correct. She admittedly stated, "You are absolutely and positively correct." I then said, while looking her straight in the eye, "Joie, you're only 21 years old. You're young and beautiful, and intelligent (I'd seen that in class). Now's the time to make your move lest you feel guilty 10 or 20 years from now. The world is yours for the taking. Let's do it together."

Joie looked at me sadly and said, "Dr. Walke, I'd give anything to because I do want too be successful. I do want to be pretty. I do so much want to be someone. But I have no money. I thought you probably knew that by my clothes and my old rickety car." She had tears in her eyes. (By the way, her financial embarrassment was just another reason I decided to put my entire program in this low-cost book. I sincerely feel this book is the best $15.00 you'll ever spend).

"I was fairly certain of that!" I answered, "But no problem. I'll do it for free on two conditions: 1) You follow my program religiously so that my time is not wasted and; 2) when you're slender and beautiful, you'll "tell them where you got it." She laughed; thanked me profusely, and we were on our way. She became one of the better—possibly the best—client I've ever had. She even gave me permission to use her actual name in this book but I decided not to.

When we began, Joie was a 5'6" young woman and weighed 245 lbs. By her own admission, she was a "tub of lard" and despised herself continually for being one. She ate everything in sight and fit every characteristic of the foodaholic that I detailed in the beginning of this book—including using food as her main sexual act (again, by her own admission). She consciously considered suicide often and knew that her eating habits were HER WAY of doing so.

I must admit that I was even more conscientious and caring in my work with Joie than usual—though I try to be close with every counselee. There was a strong aura of empathy and "good vibes" from the beginning. I don't know exactly why but have surmised since that it was due to her excellent friendly personality and the fact that she so reminded me of Diane, my aforementioned favorite cousin who LITERALLY ate herself to death at 31. In any event, Joie and I became closer than most effective counselor-counselee relationships by necessity do. I loved her—and still do—in the truest sense of one human being loving another. You need read nothing else into it.

From the very beginning, Joie practiced her tri-lateral programming fastidiously. She took her pills punctually and it was easy to observe that she was highly motivated toward success. My approach to her had been just the trigger mechanism that she needed and I was certain that I had unleashed a human dynamo who would desire much more success and achievement than just weight-loss. She was without work at the time though she once had done some sales work and some small-cabaret singing. In her words, "My lack of self-image, self-confidence, and my weight made me fail in both."

I sensed during the first few weeks that Joie was to be SOMEONE SPECIAL in my program. She soaked up ALL my principles like a sponge. And when, during the eighth week, we began discussing the WALKIAN FORMULA FOR CERTAIN SUCCESS, she actually became excited—especially since she was already well into "mysterious" thoughts and actions and was seeing some results in weight loss and body definition. I do a lot of role-playing in my counseling. Role playing with food approach; role playing with modes and styles of eating; role playing with human relations skills and how to practice them; role playing in how to be creative (coming up next); etc. Role playing in most everything discussed in this book. Joie approached her role playing like a professional actress. She literally poured herself into this "make-believe" better than any counselee I've ever had. I knew then that she was a "can't miss" person in anything she wished to do. I thought to myself, "Get your children off the streets, world, here comes Joie Koch!" A beautiful, highly-motivated "Frankenstein" was being created—there was absolutely no doubt in my mind about it.

She meticulously followed my every recommendation on symbolic eating. She was, at the end of the six weeks, already well into an enjoyable exercise regimen and a small portion diet program with no refined sugar, no grease, salt substitute, mega-vitamin dosages, and low carbohydrates.

She was already practically begging me to start her sessions with Angee. Usually I do not do so until I'm reasonably certain that one has moved past the self-discipline stage into the internalized change of approach to food stage (remember my example of peanut butter cookies in the first part of this book?). Most people do not reach this stage until almost the end of my program (approximately four months) and many persons take about a year—a few people even two years—to make the full change from "living to eat" to "simply eating to live." Remember, if you're searching for miraculous instant cures, good luck! But Joie was an exception and she began to also meet with Angee after eight weeks.

Part of Joie's mysterious thinking had to do with unusually crooked teeth. She had always been extremely self-conscious regarding them, but had never sought help from an orthodontist. In fact, she had always feared doing so. One day, following a special session I gave, she informed me that she was going to call an orthodontist immediately—and she did. That special presentation, which is an integral part of my program, is entirely built around the following universal truth:

"THE QUALITY OF LIFE YOU LIVE FROM THIS MOMENT UNTIL YOU DIE IS DIRECTLY RELATIVE TO HOW WELL YOU ARE ABLE TO DEVELOP YOUR SELF-CONCEPT AND THUS HOW HIGHLY YOU REGARD YOURSELF."

That entire presentation had special significance to Joie. She told me that not only had she not liked her unusual tooth formation, but also had not liked herself for being fearful of correcting it. She further stated that this change was just as important to her as her weight loss. Angee and I wholeheartedly agreed! She had successful oral surgery and was fitted for braces.

The entire Joie Koch story had a wonderful storybook ending—or should I say storybook BEGINNING since Joie is now only 23½ years old; a slim, trim svelt 120 lbs.; a flat-out "knock out" in almost any beholder's eyes—and a woman who dresses with simple class and wears her make-up flawlessly. Furthermore, she is pursuing (and reaching) goals she never dreamed of 2½ years ago and is setting new goals continually. AND ANYONE OF YOU CAN DO EXACTLY WHAT JOIE HAS DONE!!

She has followed most all of Angee's and my recommendations on dress and make-up for women and I wish to share them with you. Before I do, let me say that I've always seemed to have good instincts about what looks good on women. That is to say, when I select an outfit for a woman, MOST other men AND WOMEN will find that outfit very complimentary, also. When I don't like a given garment or garment combination, MOST other men and women don't approve of it on that person either. However, I do readily admit that I'm not very competent in dressing women FOR OTHER WOMEN in the world of commerce and industry. Therefore, I leave that to Angee.

HOW TO BE A BEST DRESSED WOMAN

Following are a select few of my tips on dressing well and grooming nicely for women. Some of them are Angee's, also, and they are not in any special order of priority. I consider Angela Y. Whitt a co-author on the remainder of this chapter.

A) It is even easier for women to be well-dressed and appear as though "you never wear the same outfit twice" because of the many and wonderful ACCESSORIES you can wear. Far too many women make the error of SELDOM wearing these accessories. They include such things as hats, headbands, hairbands, earrings, scarves, belts, jewelry, and high heels. I'll discuss each briefly later.

B) There is little or no excuse for a woman not being VERY well-dressed. First of all, it can be done inexpensively and secondly, there is too much information available on how to dress properly—and cheaply. Lack of money is no excuse for being a poorly dressed woman though many women rationalize their unkemptness by saying, "I could look nice, too, if I had her money. (Yet many of the women they envy shop at Goodwill and yard sales. I'm serious!) Those unkempt women are only showing poor self-image and/or ignorance. By the way, "ignorance" is a misunderstood term. When one is called "ignorant," he usually interprets that as being called dumb, silly, stupid or some similar adjective. We would understand the definition of 'ignorance" much better if we spelled it as it should be: "Ignore-unt." Ignorant means you are ignoring the vast amount of evidence, information, and knowledge that we have gathered on the subject on which you are being labeled "ignorant." Do not ignore the fact that classy dressing can be done very cheaply.

C) The same is true of women's make-up. There is no excuse for not being able to wear make-up properly. There are too many education programs (from speakers in department stores to books to pamphlets, etc.) for any woman not to have a working knowledge of the use of make-up to magnify her strengths and to cover her flaws—or at least lessen her flaws.

Most women either wear too much or too little make-up. It is so tragic to see a woman with make-up of any type "caked" on her face and it is equally embarrassing to be able to see (on the neck or top forehead) where the regular skin leaves off and the make-up begins. That woman is already exhibiting a distinct lack of knowledge and taste. A "mask" appearance is humiliating.

D) The lighter the skin, the lighter the base and vice versa. Oily skin, use water base. Dry skin, use oil base, generally speaking.

E) With blush, rose "natural" colors are preferred by most men and other women viewing you. Only use enough to highlight the cheekbones and to give you some color. Men are usually turned off badly by a "clown face." But look around you—you'll see them often every day.

F) Regarding eye shadow. As far as I'm concerned, it should be omitted entirely unless you are an actress or model appearing before camera or on stage. Eyes can be accented beautifully with mascara and eyeliner (only under bottom lashes). There's no such thing as ugly eyes.

But if you insist upon eye shadows, please stick to light natural earth tones, don't "cake" it on (ugly!), and keep the shadow limited to the lids only—not up into the eye socket!

G) Lipsticks. Small, thin lips can be made to appear larger—only by the use of darker colors, not necessarily red. But don't wander TOO much, and don't put it on too thick, even if that is the "in" look in a given year. Which brings up an important point: NEVER LET STYLE EXPERTS LEAD YOU AWAY FROM WHAT IS YOU! This practice is especially abused by women "experts," both in make-up and hairstyles—and in clothes. Coordinate your lipstick with your blush (rose and rose, peach with peach, etc.).

H) Hairstyles are just as important—possibly even more so—as your style of dress. They are the basis of everything. Most women become attached to one hairstyle and to the length of their hair. That would be like wearing the same hat every day for years. Experiment with variety and change. Again, don't worry about what's the latest fad. Dorothy Hamill, Barbara Streisand, Farrah Fawcett or Cheryl Tiegs do not look like you (probably) and they should not be dictating your hairstyle. That would be as silly as me stating in the first part of this book that every woman should weigh 103 pounds because Natalie Wood did and every man 180 pounds because I do.

Your style should feel good on you and should make you feel freer and sexier. Personally, I prefer hair long enough to give you flexibility and variety. For example, hair you can wear in various permanents; in a bun on top or in back; in a pony-tail, etc. But both Angee and my beautiful daughter, Katharine, currently have very short hair and look great. So long as it's you!

LET'S TALK
CLOTHES AND ACCESSORIES!

Since I make no pretense of being a style expert (and you needn't be either), but DO have good instincts about what men (and most women) like to see on you, I'm going to keep this very simple. Before I begin, let me say that it should go without saying that you should accent your sexual features (no matter your age—show me a woman who doesn't like feeling a little sexy and intriguing, and I'll show you a woman who is either dead or shouldn't be reading this book—or both) and camouflage your lack of them. "IF YOU'VE GOT IT, FLAUNT IT!"—at least within reason and taste. Ha, I fully realize you don't wear a bikini to your husband's funeral or a wedding dress to an orgy!

HOW TO BE ON
THE "BEST DRESSED" LIST IN
MOST AREAS FOR $600 - $800

Let me present a very frugal way that you can gain an excellent reputation as a top dresser; appear to never wear the same outfit twice; and do so over a short period of time for relatively little money. Keep in mind that A) I'm a great believer in mix 'n match in which you seldom purchase an outfit that doesn't coordinate with many others and, B) there are excellent bargains to be had in all clothes if you shop around a while. And you would be amazed how often you can buy like-new, fashionable outfits for $2.00 at yard sales, if you are patient and selective.

SPECIAL NOTE: TRUE STORY

I've watched the starlets and models who shop the most exclusive shops and look like a "million bucks." Within the past year, Angee and I have walked Fifth Avenue in New York. We've been to Beverly Hills and hob-nobbed at the exclusive clubs, including the Beverly Hills Hotel. We've been to all the casinos in Atlantic City and Las Vegas. We've walked, dined, and theatered on the mainline of Philly. We've met with the top politicians of *three states. We've been to Rio DeJaniero, Sao Paulo, and Vittoria, Brazil. Not only did Angee NEVER look or feel out of place; not only was she just as well-dressed and attractive as any woman we met; but many, many, men and women "gushed" all over her and her clothes (even wanting her to model in them!) And, so help me God, she didn't have over $900.00 in all the clothes she wore during that period. And she still wears them and will continue to—in different combinations. She's uncanny—and you can do the same!*

Just for the sake of making my point, let's say right now that you go to various stores and purchase a complete red outfit (you might personally want some design, but let me make my case). So, EVERYTHING red! First, a nice sporty or jaunty red hat of some type. Then a very low cost red headband and/or hairband. Then red earrings of some style; a red sweater styled to your body strengths; red blouse; red slacks styled to you; red skirt which shows off or covers your legs as need be; a red scarf; red belt; and red high heels. If you're in no hurry, and shop methodically over the next few weeks, you'll be astounded how "cheaply" you can accomplish all this. If I'm lying, I'm dying, I saw Angee do it last year for $67.00 but you should count on $150.00 as your target. (I can hear my beautiful and affluent readers laughing right now. Remember, affluent readers, anytime you wish to "style"—no matter how beautiful you are—in front of 500 men picked at random, and then let them rank both you and Angee's over-all appearance, I'll wager $1,000 you can't beat her. So as not to offend you, at best you'll tie. Furthermore, I'll match her $1.87 homemade bikini against your $187.00 Gucci any ole time you're ready!) CLOTHES DO NOT NEED TO BE EXPENSIVE TO BE BEAUTIFUL AND SEXY! My daughter shopped in Goodwill for years, did a little amateur sewing, and always looked like a New York model (when she wished to—Katharine was also very Bohemian, a child of the '60's).

Now, purchase the exact same complete outfit, let us say, in all white, navy blue, black, grey, and any other color which you think is "you" (pink, green, brown, beige?). You're going to do this over a period of time. That is, you're going to carefully and methodically (and simply) build a super wardrobe. If you have your head together and organize yourself, you'll have no problem.

Now it's coordinating and mix 'n match time. You know how to do it. Are you ready for this? Assume for a moment that all six outfits coordinate with each other (which, of course, they won't completely), you have the potential of literally "millions of outfits." Therefore, only a very stupid, vain or "highbrow" woman can ever say, "But I have nothing to wear." And aren't those false sophisticates so borrrrriiiinng? We even have a small group of them in Portsmouth—and they only exist in their aloof, make-believe world.

I realize I'm leaving out coats, gloves, formal wear, specialized sportswear, etc. But I've made my point. And Angee, Joie Koch, and many of my other clients are practicing this philosophy at this very moment—quite successfully.

HATS ON WOMEN

Women "miss the boat" here more than any other place. They look super in hats and most men and other women like them in hats very much. I have conducted this little study five times. I get two pictures of the same woman. In both pictures, the same woman is wearing the exact same outfit—except in one picture she has selected some type of jaunty hat, sporty hat, car cap, greek sailor cap, you name it, which matches her outfit in color and style. Then I go out and randomly poll 500 men—of all ages, race, size, and type. I keep both pictures hidden and give them these careful instructions: "When I hold up these two pictures, I want you to take a quick glance and tell me which woman is the most intriguing, the sexiest, and the one you would most want to date IF you had to date one of them. Keep in mind that I want your first reaction to her." Combining my five studies—2,500 men—a whopping 81% picked the women with hats. That's one hell of a significant number, sufficient in my mind to tell women they had better be paying attention to their hat wardrobe and selection.

And the pictures weren't just of "sexy" outfits. For example, I showed 500 randomly selected men two pictures of Angee in her nursing outfit in the exact same informal pose and asked them to give their five-second "gut" reaction as to which one they thought was most beautiful, sexy and which one they'd most like to go out with on a date. In one picture, Angee was without her nursing cap—in the other she was wearing it pertly on her head. 83% of those men selected the picture with the cap! Bareheaded women, you might wish to re-connoiteur your position. Hats add class. Class breeds success. And success breeds success! That says it all.

Headbands and hairbands are also highly effective within certain groundrules. I have always liked headbands on women. Indian braided headbands are best, though a designer kerchief, tightly-rolled, can be used nicely. The headband can be worn both across the forehead and UNDER the hair or across the forehead and OVER the hair. Both are different looks. Headbands are highly provocative to most men (I'll prove this in a moment) as they usually give the woman a "WILD INDIAN PRINCESS LOOK!" For this reason, headbands should not be worn in business or informally—only for evening wear or sportswear. The major groundrule to follow here is that no woman over forty should wear headbands unless she has that extremely rare commodity that can pass for a much younger woman. Nothing is more of a "turn-off" to most men AND OTHER WOMEN than an older woman attempting to look VERY young—an old squaw attempting to capture princess-ness again. And that is just what a headband will do! So headbands are definitely for younger women or at least women who appear younger.

The second groundrule is closely related to the first. If you are unfortunate enough to be in your late twenties or early thirties but look a little older, you should probably avoid headbands for the same reason as above. Don't ever be caught as an old hen trying to look like a young chick. It's embarrassing to you. (To appease any feminist readers, the same is true of men. Old codgers humiliate themselves by trying too hard too look like young "studs").

I also conducted careful research on headbands and the results were staggering. I picked five attractive women ranging from 19 to 35. I took pictures of them in the same outfits with identical poses and facial expressions. One picture was with headband, one without. I gave them the same "gut" reaction test already described to 500 randomly selected men. 91% (455) selected the picture WITH the headband!

However, a word of caution. Headbands are not for women who wish to be "womens' women." I polled 500 randomly selected women and gave them the five-second test as to which woman they would most want for a friend? Only 22% selected the headband picture. You see, beautiful young Indian maidens have always been a threat to both squaws and OTHER young Indian maidens—beautiful or not-so-beautiful.

Keep in mind that you change your look significantly by wearing the headband outside the hair or inside. So, that choice alone gives you two almost completely different outfits.

HAIRBANDS are different because they can be worn quite stylishly by women of ANY age—from five to 95. My definition of a hairband is one which travels from under the back of the hair vertically to the top of the head. It might tie there in a bow or be tied at the bottom with just the band showing on top. While it is true that the hairband may not be "you," it is also true that most women look very, very nice in them if style and color are carefully selected and matched. ALL women should at least give them a trial to add variety (and possibly classiness and sexiness) to their wardrobe.

SCARVES

Scarves are fantastic instruments for adding different looks to your limited wardrobe because they can be used in so many ways. For example, a large scarf is almost a semi-shawl. Therefore, it can be worn around the neck so that it dangles down the front of your outfit; or down the back; or over the shoulder. With proper pinning, they are super-stylish. Furthermore, they can be worn as bandero-type belt which is really sharp. Be creative with your scarves. The possibilities are almost limitless. And, mathematically speaking, they add a large number of outfits to your wardrobe.

JEWELRY

Earrings, necklaces, bracelets, rings, pendants, etc., are all important. They're attractive and can be bought relatively cheap. In my opinion, expensive jewelry is completely unnecessary, silly, and gaudy. Leave it for the filthy rich. I guess they have money to burn. Also, keep your jewelry simple and tasteful. I fully realize that Sammy Davis, Jr. or Cher—because of their fame—can get by with wearing rings on every finger; heavy ostentatious necklaces; bracelets all over the arm; and bright large earrings. But let's tell it like it is: Most of us think it looks stupid. The "gypsy" look or the "diamonds-are-a-girls-best-friend look" is just a turn-off to most people. It's just TOO MUCH—too over-done! Mr. "T" would be laughed at in most social situations—if we both were not so afraid of him. I guess he can wear whatever he darn well pleases.

HIGH HEELS

If I were a woman, first of all I'd never be caught in PUBLIC with complete "flats." No matter how tall or short a woman is, "flats" in ANY style of shoe—even in sandals—gives a look so negative I can't even describe it. I meet very few men who don't agree. Secondly, high heel shoes CAN be comfortable if selected and fitted well and if you physically train yourself properly.

Thirdly, if you can't wear "spike" heels all the time in public—which most of you can't—keep in mind that there are many types of elevated heels built quite comfortably. But at least wear shoes with some type of full heel, half-heel or plain heel. Believe me on this. For whatever reason, shoes are one of the most important garments a woman wears. Both men and other women will soon and quickly "check out your feet." Why? I don't know, maybe it's Freudian, but they WILL.

And make no mistake. I'm right about my discourse above on heels. I conducted my picture test, my "gut" reaction sexual test, on 500 men. In this test, one picture was of women in high heels, one without. All else was the same. ONLY TWO selected the picture with flats. That amounts to about 99 44/100%. And when I asked 50 women employers which one they would hire, 42 selected the woman with high heels. And I might add that four of the women that picked the "flats" outfit were very short in stature. It would appear to me that the "threat factor" was at work here—a tip for you in future job interviewing.

Just last evening, I attended Shawnee State's Commencement. A good many of the women wore flats or sandals with their caps and gowns. I suppose they were doing so in the name of comfort. But that makes no sense because 1) a commencement is basically a formal event; 2) one spends most of the time sitting; 3) most everyone gets his/her picture taken at least once—usually more; 4) many important people are consciously or unconsciously making judgements of you whether you (or they) know it or not; and 5) the women in flats and sandals looked like goonie little (or big) penguins flapping across the stage while the women in heels looked regal and classy. 'Nuff said. Except that women should attempt—over a period of time—to develop as complete a wardrobe in high heel shoes as possible. That is, as many different colors as is feasible so that matching shoe color with various blouses, sweaters, hats, scarves, and earrings is possible at all times. SHOES ENHANCE YOU IMMENSELY! Go to the bank on it (literally!).

TWO QUICK CASE STUDIES

I just want to present two brief cases of women with whom I'm well acquainted. They are classics to make my point on the importance of dress in women. I hope I do not offend either of them because they are two of my favorite people.

1) GAYE

Gaye (not her real name) is probably our closest female friend. Actually, we have never quite had the nerve to tell her what I'm about to write here. She will be reading this book and, of course, will know to whom I'm referring. But I do not mind because the following is a prime example of CONSTRUCTIVE CRITICISM—as both Angee and I love her very much.

First of all, Gaye is the most beautiful woman over 40 that I've ever seen—with the exception of a few Hollywood stars who have been carefully cared for, plus often having their own plastic surgeons. Hell, I'd look like Burt Reynolds right now if I had my own "molder."

Gaye's beauty still even equals most of those Hollywood beauties. In fact, her facial features and slender, lithe body are so stunning that she attracts men wherever she goes even with her "highly questionable" wardrobe. Beauty conquers about anything, doesn't it? Gaye is one of the few women one sees in her late 40's who attracts even teen-age and young adult males! But Gaye simply does not know how to dress very well. Naturally, she's always clean and pert, but her clothes are just not "her." They are often sloppy and sagging and simply do not "become" her or display her great strengths. QUITE FRANKLY, MY YOUNG, BEAUTIFUL DAUGHTER, KATHARINE MARIE, FITS MUCH THE SAME PATTERN!!

Gaye's lack of proper dress is very understandable. By her own admission, she is a country girl who spent most of her life being a mother (and a darn good one, you can bet). Therefore, she simply has had no exposure to proper and classy dress. Hypothetically, if she would just "turn herself over" to Angee and permit her to completely select her clothes, accessories, hairstyle, and make-up, Gaye would rival any woman you see on TV or movies. And there would be almost nothing she could not achieve. Men would stand in line to work for her success. They stand in line for her now—but most of the time, I fear, for a different reason!

2) BESS

Bess is a completely different case. While Bess (not her real name) is highly beautiful in her features, she is somewhat overweight and would benefit from my program. Oh, how she would look if slender! Though I suspect that her mindset will never permit her to be.

However, Bess is a highly competent librarian who does seem to have adequate self-concept and definitely knows how to dress. She has selected a tasteful and classy mode of dress which minimizes her heftiness and magnifies her beauty. She's a prime example of dressing properly—though she still needs to get her eating habits under control. Bess is possibly one of the top five classiest dressers I've seen in southern Ohio.

CONCLUSION

If you do not realize that the manner in which you dress and groom yourself is highly indicative of how much success you'll probably achieve, then you are quite foolish. If you do not understand that your mode of dress and grooming reflect your self-concept, then you are ingore-unt. If you do not comprehend that your dressing and grooming dictate how MOST people see you and relate to you, then you are playing games with yourself. HOW YOU DRESS AND GROOM WON'T AUTOMATICALLY MAKE YOU SUCCESSFUL, BUT EVEN IF YOU ARE TALENTED AND CREATIVE, SLOVENLY HABITS WILL PROBABLY KEEP YOU FROM BEING SUCCESSFUL!

THE
RODNEY DANGERFIELD SYNDROME

Before we move on to the next chapter, it seems appropriate here to discuss the word "respect." I get so many people—both men and women—who complain that they just don't get the respect they'd like from their children, spouse, boss, friends, associates, colleagues, etc. They always ask the same question, "How can I command or demand more respect?"

And my answer is always the same. "You can't!" Respect, by its very definition, cannot be commanded or demanded. Only "fear" can be commanded or demanded through intimidation and only a fool believes that "fear" and "respect" are the same. Respect, by definition, must be EARNED! Therefore, if a given person doesn't respect you, then you, at least in their eyes, have not earned it. So, the question is, "how do you EARN respect from those around you?"

Furthermore, you are in error if you think that "popularity" and "respect" are the same thing. I have many people whom I like very much—but do not respect. I also know many people that I respect—but I don't really like them at all. The same is true of me. I can name many people who do not like me (believe me!), but they prove by their daily actions that they respect me. Ideally, it is nice to have people who both like you and respect you. But, given a forced choice, I'd much rather have others respect me than like me. I don't live my life to win popularity contests. And I've learned that those who do usually lead confining and shallow lives.

So, how do you earn the respect of MOST of those people with whom you come into daily contact. As usual, the formula for doing so is quite simple. But implementing it is all up to you. Here it is:

COMPETENCE

Knowing what the heck you're doing! This takes hard work and preparation.

plus

CONFIDENCE

Knowing that you know what the heck you are doing! This takes practice and repetition.

plus

SELF-RESPECT

Including pride in personal appearance. You truly must like who you are and what you are all about.

plus

TREATING PEOPLE RIGHT

This includes common courtesy, human relations skills, fairness, and justice.

equals

AUTOMATICALLY EARNED RESPECT!

CHAPTER FOURTEEN

F) Creativity—The Final Step Toward Becoming Successful and More Fully Human

The cerebral cortex of the human brain contains from ten to twelve billion thinking cells. No other animal on earth even comes close to our brain mass and brain power. We also know that we use only a relatively small percentage of those brain cells within our lifetime. ANY NORMAL PERSON CAN BE HIGHLY CREATIVE. And not to attempt to be highly creative is to give up most of your humaneness. You then reduce yourself toward the other primates and, in fact, toward all the animals on the earth who simply exist—and exist mainly on instinct.

But when one mentions (or hears) the word "creativity," most people think that it consists of sophistication such as painting a picture, sculpting, writing a novel or song, or being a famous inventor. But these are only a few examples of creativity. It is much simpler than that and, I contend, most any human can be very, very creative. In addition, one can be creative in any aspect of life—from business to teaching and from the ministry to social work. To stretch a point there are creative bank robbers and non-creative bank robbers.

You see, creativity is simply taking known knowledge and placing it in different sequences to produce "new" knowledge. It's nothing more than that—and anyone can do it. For example, I know many men and women who are very average (or below) in native intelligence who are highly creative in developing their business and advertising schemes. There are many mechanics, housewives, and proverbial garbage collectors who are highly creative in their work and lives. And you can be also! Not to be is to limit, and even cripple, your short stay on this earth. In addition, creating and playing games with your cerebral computer is fun and challenging—once you learn how to be creative on an organized basis. SUCCESSFUL PEOPLE ARE CREATIVE PEOPLE. And they have fun playing creative games with their mind. You should set aside a part of your EVERY day to CREATE! Let me give you my favorite ways to do it and you can "borrow" or "steal" them if you wish.

A) "IDEA-TIME" (DEEP THINKING)

It is surprising (and shocking) how many people will "poke fun" when you tell them you are an "idea man" (person). There is much anti-intellectualization among grass roots people because they are threatened by thinkers and truthseekers. It has been thus ever since man became AWARE of his thinking abilities (abstract thinking). These anti-idea persons must ever be reminded of one important fact:

NOT ONE THING HAS EVER BEEN ACCOMPLISH-ED NOR HAS ONE DOLLAR EVER BEEN MADE UN-TIL SOMEONE CAME UP WITH AN IDEA!

Creative ideas are worth money. Therefore, creativity is at a premium. I never give my ideas free-of-charge unless to a friend and I try to never cast my pearls before swine—though I often do so and regret it later. You should attempt to follow the same guidelines. If you told me right now that you could show me how to profit $25,000 this year that I otherwise could not make, but that you would expect me to give you $2,250 of it. I'd be very foolish not to do so, wouldn't I. Well, you wouldn't believe how many people would refuse such an offer and will attempt to get those ideas from you without remuneration. A fool and his ideas are soon parted. Ask the inventor of the socket wrench. It almost happened to him. Ask Willie Nelson when "they" took his classic songs from him for $50 and made a fortune from them. Better still, ask me. One year ago I created a multi-million dollar idea as to how to almost completely eliminate the national shoplifting problem. But because of my lack of scientific knowledge and legal know-how, you will soon see that idea implemented world-wide and I'll realize nothing for it. Like I said, "A fool . . ."

Obviously, any time of the day one can come up with a good idea. And that idea should always immediately be written down if possible. But we know beyond a shadow of a doubt that, in most people, the brain is the most creative when it is relaxed. The more relaxed, the more creative! This is not to say that one can't create under pressure. We can prove that there are people who do. But people who can create well under pressure are people who basically can remain RELAXED under pressure (or if you please, THREAT).

Keeping this relaxation factor in mind, I have found that I come up with most of my good ideas in the morning when I awaken. Therefore, the SE-COND (note that I said "second") thing I do when I awaken in the morning is to lie still for 15 minutes, contemplating my life and present goals and recording on a bedside pad the various related ideas that come to me. I've had many great ones, and some mornings my brain is so fruitful that I cannot believe the number of goodies it bears. The note pad is essential lest you become frustrated that you might not be able to recall them all, and thus your mind becomes jumbled. If you put knowledge into your brain (learning), it is astounding what it "spits out" later in the realm of creativity, if you create on an almost daily, organized basis.

I then proceed to the shower and spend another highly-relaxed ten minutes in "idea-time." Again, many of my best ideas through the years have been while showering. So, thus far, I've spent approximately 25 minutes already in creative thinking time. But you will remember I stated that "idea-time" was the second thing I do upon awaking. The FIRST is also creative time—and I'll wager you have overlooked it. Please do not do so any longer.

B) DREAMS

Most people don't realize just how creative dreams are and/or do not know how to tap this great free-flowing fountain of creativity. The human brain is most relaxed when you are asleep. It literally is running free and thoughts just race from conscious (recall) to unconscious (can't recall) and vice versa. The brain is virtually "at play" and having a grand ole' time—whether the particular dream is a fantasy (wish-fulfillment) one or an anxiety (nightmare) one, or somewhere in between. Dreams are the ultimate example of creativity purely defined. The brain is taking known information and re-working it into new patterns. MANY OF OUR MOST CREATIVE PEOPLE HAVE DERVIED SOME OF THEIR MOST NOTED CREATIONS FROM THEIR DREAMS! This is fact and it has been repeatedly noted and documented. I assure you that some of my better ideas have come from my dreams and the dream "brainstorming" I do IMMEDIATELY upon awaking.

Here is my procedure and I highly recommend it to you. The FIRST thing I do when I awaken in the morning is to record on my bedside note pad all that I can remember of my dreams. I then take approximately 10 minutes to "brainstorm" those dreams. (I'll explain my brainstorming technique in the next section). It is great fun and often highly productive (even monetarily lucrative) to brainstorm your dreams. So, you see, I have spent approximately 35 minutes of creative thinking time even before I've gone to work—and it has been at the time of day when one's mind is best suited for creativity. Try it, you'll like it.

I can think of at least three major creative ideas which have brought much success and/or money to business men to whom I've served as consultant that came directly from my dreams and the subsequent brainstorming of them upon awakening.

C) BRAINSTORMING

Some of the greatest and most positive changes of my life have taken place as a result of this simple little brain game I've learned to play. Of course, I didn't invent it and it's nothing new, but you should play it, also. It is the ultimate in HUMANNESS—that is, the daily use of your awesome cerebral brain mass—your computer. I've emphasized this often (probably over-kill) in this book, I know, but your potential and your ability to change must be imprinted deep into your own mind.

I brainstorm often with many ideas but let me give you a true example of how I brainstormed a dream and made a lot of money for a close friend of mine who had just bought a restuarant—his first business venture. The restaurant was located on a high-traffic highway but was semi-hidden down in an incline. My friend was on a "shoestring." He had indebted himself to the hilt and the entire venture was now "bootstrap." The restaurant's clientel had dwindled badly but my friend did have a background in the food-service field and knew how to serve quality food. However, his knowledge of advertising and promotion was nil and void. Since I do a lot of consulting in this area, I agreed to help him FREE—on one condition. He had to trust my judgment and use all my ideas. I've learned my lesson about casting pearls before swine! If I'm going to create free-of-charge then I at least expect those ideas to be used so that I am able to see the fruits of my labor as compensation. That seems reasonable, does it not?

The very night of our verbal agreement, I had a fascinating anxiety dream (moderate nightmare). I learned long ago not to fear my dreams. They are to be welcomed because of the creative opportunity they may afford you. I urge you to take the same viewpoint. In this particular wild and crazy dream (which most are) I was in Las Vegas walking the "Strip" viewing the neon extravaganzas and was not able to find my way back to my hometown of Jackson, Ohio. I had to be at work in my parents' grocery store and I simply could not get out of Las Vegas. Many of you have probably had a similar type dream. We call them "punctuality-anxiety" in dream classification.

Most dreams take place in REM (rapid eye movement) sleep—when you are beginning to waken—so I was soon awake and recording this simple short dream. Then I "brainstormed" it. There are many different styles of brainstorming, but here is mine:

A) I begin with the ground rule that no idea is too far out or outlandish. There is little sense in turning 10-12 billion thinking cells loose if you are going to place restrictions on them. "Fire at will, Gridley!"

B) I clearly define both in my mind and on paper the problem to be solved or the goal to be achieved. For example, in the case of my friend's restaurant, the goal (and problem) was simply to somehow stop HIS SHARE of cars from the busy highway; get the drivers into his establishment; get their billfolds off their hips or out of their purses; feed them quality food and drink within a classy atmosphere; and thereby entice them to return.

C) I look at the idea (in this case, the dream) and begin "free association" to the tune of five words—each word the first that pops into my mind after repeating the previous word. I then copy those five words down on paper.

D) Now comes IMMEDIATE SYNTHESIS. By this, I mean that I quickly take all five of those words and encompass them into one unified idea that will solve the problem or reach the goal. Remember, I am simply unharnessing my mind and no idea is considered too wild, crazy, or "far out" during the synthesis stage. I will usually repeat the free association and synthesis stage at least five times, usually ten, and oftentimes far more repetitions if time permits. Naturally, each brainstorming example is recorded as I go.

E) EVALUATION; FEASIBILITY, AND IMPLEMENTATION

After completing the steps above, I will usually wait a few hours or a few days to evaluate the feasibility of my brainstormed ideas. Are they rational and logical? Are they realistic? What is the cost? Do they fit the image and goals of the person or business to whom I'm recommending them? More often than not, the answers to these questions are "no" because brainstorming is such a cerebral "Chinese fire drill." I've often stated that 99% of my ideas are hairbrained. Ah, but when the answer is "yes," then my whole day is made—and usually some money is made, also. You see, it's that 1% that I'm hunting for. Let me give you an example by relating my brainstormed ideas for my friend's restaurant. Keep in mind that a) it came from my Las Vegas-hometown dream, and b) I created this idea on ONLY MY THIRD brainstorming idea—a total time period of about FOUR minutes.

My five completely free association words (with my personal explanation) were:

1. Marquee (self-explanatory, emanating from the Las Vegas Strip.)

2. Billboards (still self-explanatory).

3. Large (still self-explanatory, if you've been there).

4. Bill Gunn (a man who had once built a home-made large marquee for me when I was managing my family's grocery store a decade ago during my late Father's illness).

5. Make money. (Bill Gunn had long been a man I admired because he was so enterprising; always worked for himself; and always knew how to "make money."

Now it was synthesis time—a highly creative, free-flowing brief period. My synthesis was to recommend that my friend build a large, brightly-lit combination marquee-billboard—larger than any in the area; to get Bill Gunn to do it because I knew Bill worked at very low-cost; and to show my friend that not only would the marquee be built FREE of charge to him, but that he would actually MAKE MONEY on the sign while advertising his wares and promoting good public relations. Heads he wins—tails he wins.

I went to him immediately. He liked the idea but exclaimed, "How on earth do I get this thing FREE and even make money?"

"Easy,' I responded, "In fact, you can have your money in hand to build it before you even start." He looked at me increduously, so I detailed the procedure for him. (I will wager that there will be at least one businessman, possibly more, who will use the following idea. Do you think he's not getting his $14.95 worth from this book?)

A) Get together with Bill Gunn and draw-up a rough sketch and blueprint of what is to be your huge (even gaudy), bright marquee—billboard combination. Get a cost estimate. Let's say it is about $3,000.00 (I was fairly certain Bill would do it for that).

B) Take those plans to your suppliers, local business and industry, local college or university, radio or TV stations, etc.

C) Inform them that for a fee (let's say $500.00 annually), you will place in giant letters across your marquee—one day a week—such advertising as "We Proudly Serve all Flowers' Baking Products" or "Ports City, Ohio, Home of WPOY Radio'' or ''Proudly The Home of Podunk University,'' etc. Therefore, on a given day, your marquee might read:

TONIGHT THE BIG BAND '40's SOUND IN OUR LOUNGE

PRIME RIB $6.95

WE PROUDLY SERVE MILLER LITE ON DRAFT.

You promote, you advertise, you make money!!

My buddy then uttered the words that any teacher likes to hear; the statement that any creative person lives for; when he said, ''Gee, I'd never thought of it that way before, Jerry!'' To make a long story short, my good friend had $3,500.00 in his pocket BEFORE he began construction. After the first year, each subsequent year that $3,500.00 was all clear profit. His business increased significantly. He is grateful. And I have the satisfaction each time I pass the sign that it was my idea. We all win. Is this just an isolated case where I happened to hit one. Are you serious? I do it all the time! And so do many other people. And so can you. My brain is no better than yours. I have just learned how to use mine. So can you. I have shown you how in this book! I call all this ORGANIZED CREATIVITY.

CREATIVITY AND RAIN

We might as well discuss another little oddity of mine regarding creativity. However, I have a feeling that many others are similar, though they may not admit it. That is, I also seem to create better when it is raining or snowing. There are probably both deep psychological and biological reasons for this relationship of water to relaxation and therefore creativity. I think this is the reason so many highly creative writers, sculptures, poets, etc. try to locate near the sea.

In my opinion, either one (or both) of the following reasons are why water and creativity go hand-in-hand with so many humans:

1) There is overwhelming evidence now that all life was once in the sea and that we evolved from water animals. Yes, not only was your great grand-daddy (with many ''greats'' attached) a fish, but even YOU once were. You lived in a bag of salt water and YOU even had gill slits.

2) When it rains, sleets or snows, man psychologically views this as a ''time-out'' period. It comes from far back in our ancestry. When it storms, everyone takes cover, including all our natural enemies down through the ages—the giant reptiles, saber-toothed tigers, wild boars, snakes, Neanderthal men, Indians, the British, Japanese, Germans, North Koreans, Vietnamese, autocratic bosses, power-hungry police, lawyers hunting for lawsuits, etc.

Therefore, we instinctively relax because our foes are not lurking about. They're heading for their caves and shelter also. Hence, creativity time!

ATTENTION STARVING ARTISTS!

Isn't it interesting that so many artists and other highly creative people can create so magnificently but then can't create ways to make money from their creations. Of course, some don't wish to, but even those who DO like monetary reward usually find difficulty in creating marketing ideas for their works.

My son, Brad, fits this stereotype so this section of my book is kind of an open letter to him (though I told him all this long ago). Brad is a very talented artist. He can even paint portraits of people which almost always look exactly like them and highly life-like. Even many noted artists through the ages have not been able to do same. It is quite a talent and gift.

But Brad also likes the finer things of life—cars, high-class restaurants, windsurfers, women, etc. Nothing wrong with that—more power to him. So long as he uses my success formula or his own, to reach those goals.

I have told him many times that making big bucks from his creations would be easy but thus far he has either always scoffed at me and/or been too complacent and comfortable to carry through the ideas. For example, our Athletic Director at Shawnee State, Harry Weinbrecht, offered Brad a tidy sum to paint a portrait of his late son, Michael, and Brad never even followed up on the offer. By the way Harry Weinbrecht and his son, who died of muscular dystrophy, are a great human interest story. Observing Harry care for his son during those final years of deterioration is one of the more beautiful experiences of valiance, love, and gallantry I've ever witnessed. God bless you for that, Harry, and "Good night, Mr. Michael-Bash, wherever you are!"

But back to artists and creative marketing. Recently, I watched a very impressive scenario in a small bar in Portsmouth. Keep in mind that the artist in this situation was at most only of above average skill; that he was in all probability an alcoholic; and that the bar is frequented usually by people of quite limited income. Also, bear in mind that Angee and I were there for approximately three hours watching an Ohio State football game.

During that time span, we watched this "artist," using only an art pencil and large drawing pad (that's called low overhead), sketch a person sitting in the bar while he (the artist) also watched the game. He would soon approach the "drawee" and show him/her the picture and asked if they'd like to purchase it for $6.00. In those three hours, he sold 14 pictures—$84.00 or $28.00 per hour. If the answer was "no," he smiled nicely and presented them with their picture free. They usually at least bought him a drink—as did the "yes" people. Free drinks, free football, and $84.00. Fairly profitable little afternoon if you ask me.

But I told you that I'm creative, also. At the conclusion of the game, I approached him and complimented his ingenuity. Then I told him that I knew how he could increase his profit 50%—that is, make $9.00 per sketch rather than six. He quickly asked me how to do so. I told him seriously that I don't give out my ideas free. He grew suspicious, of course, until I smiled and said, "Buy me a beer, and I'll tell you." He smiled in return and paid me my consulting fee.

I told him to go downtown and buy some cheap black wooden picture frames ($4.00 each at most when bought in bulk) and frame the pictures before he approached potential customers. Then charge $10.00 rather than six. By coincidence, I saw him two weeks later in another bar in our fair city. He had his little gym bag of frames; informed me that his sales had increased, even though charging $10.00; and thanked me for my idea. I work cheap, don't I? BY THE WAY, YOU CAN GO TO THE BEST PSYCHIATRIST OR WEIGHT PROGRAMS IN THE COUNTRY AND PAY HUNDREDS OF DOLLARS FOR WHAT YOU'RE GETTING HERE FOR $14.95.

A SPECIAL NOTE ON
ALCOHOL, DRUGS, AND CREATIVITY

There has been much written over the years regarding the heightened awareness, increased relaxation, and the accompanying high creativity some persons experience under the various altered states produced by drugs and alcohol. Many noted writers, actors, business persons, painters, sculpters, etc., have claimed to have some of their most productive work and/or ideas occur during drug/alcohol "highs"—or even stupors. Others adamantly state this is not so.

Obviously, I can only quote to you from my own experiences. I have already attested that MOST of my best thoughts and creations emanate from a fresh mind in the morning or during relaxed meditation during the day. I WISH TO FURTHER EMPHASIZE THAT I DO NOT PARTAKE OF ANY HARD DRUGS OR NARCOTICS—INCLUDING MARIJUANA! However, I do imbibe occasionaly in the drug of alcohol—mainly beer. I wish to again add that I do not drink very often at this time in my life. And I have had three types of experiences insofar as creativity and alcohol relate: 1) I've done some of my most creative work while on a "beer high"; 2) I've done some of my worst (dumbest) work while "high"; and 3) I've done some of my worst work and thought it was great—at the time—while "high."

Therefore, I have a groundrule I always follow: I don't do any creative work "live" while drinking. That is, no public speaking, teaching, personal appearances, etc. But I will sometimes write in rough draft or jot down ideas while "high." This allows me to clearly evaluate my creations AFTER the alcohol is out of my body system. Sometimes it's so asinine that I can't believe it came from my mind—but periodically it's pure genius, both to my now sober brain and by the evaluation of other sober minds. However, I do not recommend drugs or drink in order to create for any age group. They are just not necessary. My 10-12 billion cell computer doesn't need them. Neither does yours!

CONCLUSION

You have just read my complete formula for successful living. A chart summarizing it is on the next page. Now it is up to you to put that formula to work for yourself. Combined with your near future weight loss, and your newly-found self-concept, your life should begin to take on new depth and dimension that you had never before thought possible. It's all up to you. However, we're not quite finished yet. An extra "treat" for you follows in the next chapter as you are now prepared for EXISTENTIAL LIVING!

THE
WALKIAN FORMULA
OF
CERTAIN SUCCESS

WORK HARD

+

PLAY HARD

+

THE EIGHT BASIC HUMAN RELATIONS SKILLS

+

High Achievement   *Low Infavoidance*   *Low Abasement*
Needs   *Needs*   *Needs*

+

PRIDE IN APPEARANCE AND GROOMING

+

CREATIVITY
(Which is Easy!)

= 's

AS MUCH SUCCESS* AS YOU WISH—NO MATTER
YOUR DEFINITION OF SUCCESS

* Money? Prestige? Status? Power? Peace of Mind?
Security? Satisfaction?

CHAPTER FIFTEEN

Existential Living

You may or may not have heard of the term "Existentialism." It is mainly a philosophic school of thought made profound by the likes of Kierkegard, Tillich, Sartre, et al. But the term is also kicked around quite loosely in the field of psychology. To be honest, though many of my professors at Ohio State University 20 years ago both espoused and taught it, it was never explained to me so that I clearly understood what the heck it meant, anyway.

But now I do think I clearly know what EXISTENTIALISM is and I'm going to try to capture it for you in simple words and concepts—the essence of good teaching. And I must begin by saying three things to you: 1) The roots of Existentialism are not new. Socrates, Christ, Gandhi, Muhammed, and many other wise persons spoke many Existential philosophies. 2) However, Existentialism has really only BLOSSOMED in the past 100 years—and more specifically, in the past 30 years. 3) Most of you reading this book are much more existential than you probably realize and ALL of you are somewhat existential. It would be nearly impossible not to be in our modern, technological, mass media age.

HOW GRANDMA AND GRANDPA LIVED AND MANY STILL DO!

Naturally, throughout the long history of man's existence on this earth (there is almost irrefutable evidence that it has been three to five million years), he has spent night and day just trying to survive against his enemies (both man and beast) and against the elements (wind, rain, bacteria, pestilence, etc.).

But since the advent of the scientific age—and more particularly since the end of World War II—we in the modern nations have been "blessed" with fantastic amounts of leisure time (compared to our forefathers at least) in which to develop our intellect, creativity, recreational life, etc. Of course, like all "gifts" in life, there is always a price to pay. So we can form a legitimate argument that this vast amount of leisure time is not always a "blessing" and that it is often a "curse." Nevertheless, few people in their right minds would REALLY, TRULY wish to go back to the "good ole' days" during which people died of minor diseases and infections; one had to go out in the freezing cold to an outdoor toilet at 2:00 a.m.; it would take 20 men five days of back-breaking labor to dig a ditch that a backhoe will now dig in 15 minutes, etc. Modern science has given us the time to grow and develop far beyond any of our great grandparents—though we owe everything we are to them and the heritage they gave us.

However, that's not the point here. Nor is it the point of Existentialism. The point here is that most of our parents, most of our grandparents, most of our great-grandparents and, more importantly, MOST PEOPLE TODAY do not know how to live existentially. Therefore, they are not capable of fulfilling their humanness; of becoming more fully human; or of reaching maximum levels of potential, growth, and development.

You must understand that most of you reading this book right now, without realizing it, have not learned the psychological techniques of LIVING IN THE "NOW"—existing in the "NOW." You spend most of your waking day living in the FUTURE, being that 10 seconds from now or 10 years from now, or living in the PAST, whether 10 seconds ago or 10 years ago. Therefore, you're just "waterbugging" over the surface of the POND OF NOW rather than diving into the POND OF NOW and living a life of depth and quality. Probably right now, and understandably so, you are saying, "That's ridiculous, Jerry, of course I'm living in the "now." I'm reading this book right "now," aren't I? I'm here right "now," aren't I?"

Well, of course, you are. But I'll still wager that you're probably not a participator in existential living—or at least not nearly as much as you should be from day-to-day. Let's see if I can "prove" it to you. Let's see if I'm not correct that the following parable hits very close to how you live your life—and a near proximity to most peoples' lifestyles:

THE WILLIAM/WILHELMA JONES PARABLE

This parable could also appropriately be entitled "My life really isn't real happy NOW but when I reach THAT point in life, THEN, by gosh, I'll be happy." Because that is a pattern (trap) that many of us fall into—thinking that our life NOW really isn't so fulfilling, but some point soon, ten minutes, ten hours, ten days, ten months, or ten years from NOW, it will be. We only skip over the "POND OF NOW" rather than diving in and really "getting into it" (a classic existential phrase our youth have coined) each moment.

Little William (or Wilhelma) Jones is a nice all-American four-year-old boy (girl) in the neighborhood. You probably will recognize him (her) soon because, very possibly, he/she was once you.

William has been enjoying his free play with his peers in the neighborhood for a year or more now but is beginning to feel some discontent. Some of his "older" buddies have gone off to kindergarten now and tell him of their various and asundry experiences. So even though life in the neighborhood is still, "O. K., I guess," little William just can't wait until he, in actuality, also gets to go to school. In other words, "Life's not bad, but when I reach kindergarten, then I'll have it made, THEN I'll be happy!"

Before long, William finds himself in kindergarten. And ziiippp, right back down to the bottom rung he goes. Oh, it's O.K., that kindergarten, but it's just not all it's cracked up to be. Those boring naps on rugs, which almost any red-blooded boy with an active thyroid detests. And learning colors, numbers, shoe-tying, and other "stuff" he already knew anyway. Besides, he doesn't get to take recess at the same time as the grade schoolers—and even then has to play stupid, little kid games instead of games big boys play. Plus, the first graders get to learn reading, writing, and arithmetic and all kinds of other academic goodies. This kindergarten is just not all it's ballyhooed to be. But when he gets to be a big first-grader, THEN he'll have it made, by gosh.

So, all too soon (at least by parents' perception) little Willie is a big first grader. And you guessed it, ziiipp, back down to the bottom of the pecking order he speeds. Not that first grade is so bad, you understand, but William isn't too impressed. How can one be when now he has homework; and now he sees the kids in the upper elementary grades already knowing how to read and write; and he sees how much bigger, stronger and more sophisticated they are; and he notes that they are able to play "big boy" games at recess and relegate him to the edge of the playground for sissy games like Red Rover and Freeze Tag. Nope, this first grade scene just ain't all it's cracked up to be, buddy. "But when I get to be a big second grader, THEN I'll be O.K. And the third grade? Oh, super! And the fourth? Yeh! And the fifth and sixth graders even get to switch classes and have more than one teacher.

And they get to play little league baseball instead of "yukky" T-ball. Boy, when I get to sixth grade, THEN I'll be happy."

Well, how quickly he enters sixth grade and puberty. Whooommmppp! Back down to a sad awakening. The age of "tits and zits." The land of pimples and worrying about breasts that are too small (Wilhelma) or too big due to baby fat (William). Will anyone want to kiss him at the parties? "Why am I not big and strong like the seventh and eighth graders?" And they play organized junior high sports rather than little Little League. And they get to stay out later and hold "wilder" parties. And they go to their own school (or even down to the high school). "Gosh, sixth grade pretty much sucks! I'll be glad when I get to junior high, THEN I'll be home free.

Junior high time arrives. ZAAAPPP! Humility time at the bottom of the totem pole. Adolescence and its myriad of crucial, earth shattering problems and decisions. "Am I sexy? Do I measure up? Am I going to make the team or the cheerleading squad or the majorette corps? Will I get asked to the dance or will anyone accept my invitation? Heck, the high school kids practically run over you in the hallways. And they have real parties, and car dates, and get to stay out really late, and play VARSITY sports, and they seem so confident and poised. Junior high is the pits, man! I'll be glad when I get to high school. Man, THEN I'll truly have it made, yeah!"

Freshman year, and ole Willie begins to learn some more facts of life at the bottom of the barrel. Freshman and reserve teams rather than varsity stardom, Algebra, Latin, and American Literature. Homework galore. Parents still much too strict. Am I man enough to cut it in a man's world and woman enough to be my own woman? Those seniors are so suave. And they have their own cars. Boy, I'll be glad when I get my license. I sure "love" Jennifer, but she pays no attention to me. Will I be glad when I'm a senior. They have it made. They run the school. THEN I'll really be something. "Life now is O.K., I suppose, but THEN I'll be THE MAN!"

Much too quickly (again, as seen through Mom and Dad's eyes) William and Wilhelma are seniors. And it's almost all over, those "wonderful" school days. "I hate to leave my friends, but I'll be glad when I can get out of this school and this town. Mom and Dad still run my life too much. But when I get to college like some of my friends, that'll be the day. Independence, dorms, fraternities and sororities, partying, and adulthood. I'm tired of being treated like a kid. I'm ready to get with my life. I just can't wait to get to college. THEN, I'll have it truly made."

Good bye hometown, hello Podunk U.! And welcome to the bottom rung, Frosh! Never realized there was this much studying, did you? Are you going to make the grades. Are you going to make the team? What are you going to major in? What do you REALLY want to do the rest of your life? "Mom and Dad just aren't giving me enough spending money. They don't realize how expensive everything is." But the seniors have it made. They don't have to study as much as they've really got college life "together." "Establishing yourself in college is tough but in two or three years, THEN it will be great!"

Senior year and alma mater time. "Am I going to get a good job in my field? I'm ready to go out on my own now. I'm sick and tired of depending on Mom and Dad. I'll be glad to get out of this place, quit studying, and begin to take my place in the world. I'll have my own aparment. I'll be my own person and live a life of autonomy, success, and partying in the big city. C'mon Commencement Day. THEN, I'll commence to be happy."

William starts his first job in the computer department of A. T. and T. or as the junior high football coach at Midvale. And whew, is it hit bottom time again! "Damn, I don't even make enough money to support my family properly. I'm just a peon in the company (school). The executives (head coaches) have it made and I'll be glad when I'm one of those. THEN I'll be making a decent living. THEN, I'll be able to enjoy the fruits of life. Thank God for Friday's (future thinking again) until my ship comes in. And bills, bills, bills. I never realized how much groceries, utilities, and over-all living expenses were."

Life begins to speed up now for William and Wilhelma. The New Years Eves' and the birthdays roll around much more quickly. Soon William is a junior executive at A. T. and T. or head basketball coach at Midvale. He can't believe the pressure to produce (win). And he didn't realize how his reflexes had slowed at 35—and how gravity had taken its toll on his formerly hard stomach. And thinning hair. Yuk! "Those top executives lead the good life in their big homes, big cars, and six-figure salaries. Those college coaches like Dean Smith and Bobby Knight travel with the elite, too. They don't have to put up with the shit like we do. I'll probably never make it up there. But if I do, THEN I'll be in heaven. If not, I'll be glad when I can retire. THEN, I'll do all the things I've always wanted to do."

But wait, William, before retirement comes middle age. I'm an expert on middle-age. Let me tell you about it. First, the sure sign you are in it is when you start calculating how many GOOD years you have left and when you start hearing of acquaintances dying. If they're your own age, or younger, you feel you are living on borrowed time. If they're older, you start doing quick subtraction as to how soon it may be for you. Age spots appear; hair disappears; wrinkles appear; stamina disappears; college age children appear; money disappears; thoughts of health, nursing homes, security, wills, and cemetery plots appear; thoughts of youth, virility, and endless energy disappear. Unfulfilled goals and dreams haunt you. But, not to worry. Like you said, when you can retire, THEN you'll have it made, right?

Well, you know what usually happens. You retire and soon lose health or die. And you spent your entire life living basically in the future or in the past. You just never learned to take an existential approach to living. Below is just about how you squandered your life—and you cheated yourself. You skipped over the "NOW!"

Non-Existential Diagram

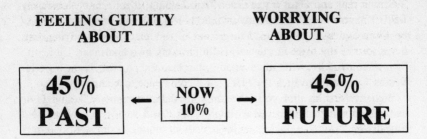

FEELING GUILITY
ABOUT

WORRYING
ABOUT

45%
PAST

NOW
10%

45%
FUTURE

Now permit me to explain the above drawing. First, keep in mind that the "future" may mean any time hence—ranging from 30 seconds from now to 30 years from now. Secondly, keep in mind that the "past" may mean any time span from 30 seconds ago to 30 years ago. Therefore, let's just say, for example, that you were sitting in a classroom daydreaming about what you were going to do after that class rather than "getting into" the class and deriving the most possible from that learning experience. Then, at least at that time, you would not be participating in existential living.

Or let's say you are spending a great deal of time feeling guilty about something you did yesterday. Non-existential living. Or possibly you worry a great deal about a test coming up tomorrow. Again, non-existential living. If you live a major portion of your life even SOMEWHAT CLOSE to the above drawing—and millions do—then you are not soaking up the NOW. You are not living one day (actually, moment) at a time as you should be. You are not living in day-tight (minute tight) compartments as you ought to be. You need to be more aware of your existence NOW (hence, EXISTEN-TIALISM!)

Existential Living Diagram

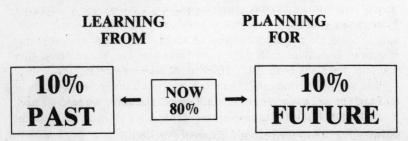

LEARNING
FROM

PLANNING
FOR

10%
PAST

NOW
80%

10%
FUTURE

On the surface, it may appear that the only difference between the drawing above and the previous diagram on non-existential living is purely semantic. That is, it may seem that my choice of wording is the only change and that such is "double-talk!" But that is not so! There is a tremendous difference in the psychological approach to life depicted in the latter diagram (existential) as opposed to the former. The existential drawing says:

"I desire to experience each moment of my existence as fully as possible. I want to "get into" EVERYTHING I undertake as much as possible—even if it's negative (such as a job you don't like). I am not interested in feeling guilty about my past actions, even if recent. And I'm further not interested in squandering time fretting and worrying about the future. I will spend a minimum amount of time, naturally, PLANNING for future events. And I'll also spend a minimal time pondering and LEARNING from my past experiences. But mostly I just want to enjoy my existence NOW on this earth—no matter the activity in which I'm presently participating."

SOME CONTEMPORARY EXISTENTIAL PHRASES

Following are some typical existential phrases that you have probably heard in TV commercials, songs, poems, etc.:

1) You only go around once in life. Do it with gusto.

2) Stop and smell the roses.

3) I really get into _____ .

4) Do your own thing.

5) Give it your best shot.

6) (Paraphrased) Don't worry about tomorrow. The lillies in the field don't and even King Solomom in all his glory wasn't arrayed as beautiful as they.

7) I gotta' be me.

8) I can't be right for somebody else if I'm not right for me (a great self-concept statement, also).

9) I did it my way!

10) For what is a man, what has he got? If not himself, then he has naught (nothing).

11) I can't be you and you can't be me. I wasn't placed on this earth to meet your expectations.

12) We all march to the beat of a different drummer.

13) It's my life and I alone am responsible for my actions. I'll live it as I choose—not as you choose.

14) You're not in the business of running other people's lives—nor am I.

15) Before I die, I want to do it all, I want to experience everything possible.

IS EXISTENTIALISM A SELFISH PHILOSOPHY BASED UPON "EAT, DRINK, AND BE MERRY, TOMORROW YOU MAY DIE?"

Although many people interpret Existentialism as described in the heading above, in its truest sense it is NOT that. The "I" or "me" generation does not, in its true form, practice a philosophy of "only my life counts and to hell with you."

Quite the contrary. Existentialism is highly UNSELFISH and most unegocentric. It simply means that my existence can have no real meaning to you IF it has little or no meaning to me. It means that my abilities to be intimate with (love) you are directly relative to my abilities to love, accept, and be intimate with myself.

It means that when I love, I love deeply; when I work, I work hard; when I play, I play spontaneously and freely; when I suffer, I suffer genuinely; when I cry, I do so unashamedly; and when I think, I think rationally, logically, intellectually, and deeply.

I have carried the following newspaper clipping in my billfold for ten years, and I read it often as a reminder: "Martin Sheen sent me a Christmas card one year with a copy of a note written by an elderly woman. In it she said if she had life to live over again, she wouldn't do any thing different except she would dance longer, stay up later, sing louder, laugh harder, cry more. Just live everything more fully. And that is just what I am trying to do."

Well, that's what Jerry L. Walke is trying to do, also. That's the essence of Existentialism. May I recommend it to you, too.

BOOK CONCLUSION

It took me about six months to write this book, but the ideas are basically a culmination of the last 15 - 20 years of my life. If it helps you lose weight and/or be successful, please write and let me know. I assure you that to help others is the major reason I wrote this book. My priorities are mostly altruistic. Any money I make is nice—but still second. Heck, I gave to charity ALL my profits from my first book.

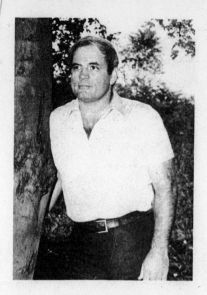

Dr. Jerry L. Walke

ABOUT THE AUTHOR

Jerry L. Walke has been a college educator for well over 20 years in various college and universities in Ohio. He was also Vice-President for Academic Affairs at Urbana College for seven of those years. He has been named to the Jaycee's "Outstanding Young Men of America" and listed in "Who's Who in American College and University Administrators." He is currently an Associate Professor of Psychology at Shawnee State College in Ohio.

Dr. Walke has an excellent reputation as a teacher, public speaker, counselor, and writer. He has a long list of client successes in the area of obesity and weight control. Jerry has held numerous seminars on weight loss—weight control for business, industry, schools, churches, etc. He has published a book, GUILT—GO TO HELL!, a wide variety of self-help booklets, and many journal articles. He is currently completing work on a textbook in human relations, two novels, and a book on parent/child relationships entitled RAISING CHILDREN FOR THE 21st CENTURY.

Jerry is himself a confirmed—and reformed—"foodaholic," having lost well over 100 pounds and maintaining same now for many years. He has become a master of teaching others the SPECIFIC techniques of losing weight, changing lifestyles, and altering self-concept. "I am not a therapist—I am a teacher, an educator," he states emphatically, and there are few people who are able to teach others the knowledge they possess as well as Jerry L. Walke. This highly unique book is a tribute to his talent for teaching and his ability to WRITE TO YOU AS THOUGH HE WERE ACTUALLY TALKING TO YOU!

Dr. Walke has also spent extensive time in Rio De Janeiro, Sao Paulo, and Vitoria, Brazil, studying the nutritional, dietary, and obesity problems of that country.

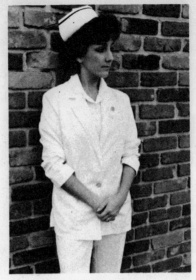

Angela Y. Whitt

ABOUT
THE COLLABORATING AUTHOR

Angela Y. Whitt is a very unique woman who has accomplished much at a young age. She is presently a registered nurse employed by the Scioto Valley Health Foundation. She currently works at Southern Hills Hospital with psychiatric care and alcohol and drug abuse. She has been working in the health care field since 13-years-old, beginning as a candy-striper and since serving as a nursing assistant, nursing technician and home care nurse.

She has also done extensive modeling in various fashion shows and for numerous department stores and agencies. In addition, she conducts seminars on how to dress and groom for success and has done private counseling and consulting in the same areas. She has displayed the unusual ability of working with both men and women as to proper and fashionable dress and grooming skills.

Ms. Whitt also specializes in diet and nutrition and is herself a vegetarian. She recently traveled to Brazil to study the renowned work of the Brazilians in the area of weight loss, weight control, and dietetics. Dr. Walke accompanied her on this fact-finding tour.